The African-American Health Book

A Prescription for Improvement

by Valiere Alcena, M.D., FACP

A Citadel Press Book
Published by Carol Publishing Group

Carol Publishing Group Edition, 1995

First published under the title *The Status of Health of Blacks
in the United States of America* by Kendall/Hunt Publishing
Company, Dubuque, Iowa, 1992.

A Citadel Press Book
Published by Carol Publishing Group
Citadel Press is a registered trademark of Carol Communications, Inc.

Editorial Offices: 600 Madison Avenue, New York, NY 10022
Sales & Distribution Offices: 120 Enterprise Avenue, Secaucus, NJ 07094
In Canada: Canadian Manda Group, One Atlantic Avenue, Suite 105
Toronto, Ontario, M6K 3E7

Queries regarding rights and permissions should be addressed to:
Carol Publishing Group, 600 Madison Avenue, New York, NY 10022

Manufactured in the United States of America
ISBN 0-8065-1719-0

10 9 8 7 6 5 4 3 2 1

Carol Publishing Group books are available at special discounts
for bulk purchases, sales promotions, fund raising, or
educational purposes. Special editions can also be created to
specifications. For details contact: Special Sales Department,
Carol Publishing Group, 120 Enterprise Ave., Secaucus, NJ 07094

The Cataloging-in-Publication Data for this title may be obtained
from the Library of Congress.

Contents

Acknowledgments

I would like to dedicate this book to the memories of—

My mother, Florisane Lacoste, who died giving birth without receiving any medical attentions.

To my father, Lamartine Alcena, who died from a perforated peptic ulcer without receiving any medical attentions.

To my children Juanita, Marcette, Valerie, Reynolds and Kevin.

To Rosalyn Sandberg, who helped organize and transcribe the first eight chapters of this book prior to her death. She was a most precious human being.

To my friend Karen Allison, M.D. who kept me encouraged while writing this book.

To Dr. Ana Paulino for her help in organizing the manuscript.

To several of my physician colleagues at White Plains Hospital Medical Center who provided me with several of the photographs used in this book.

Preface

Black Americans are sicker than their white counterparts.

Blacks in this country are affected more by every disease than whites. The reasons for these discrepancies are:

1. Blacks are poorer than whites and have less money for good medical care.
2. The level of achieved education among Whites is higher than Blacks; consequently, Blacks have less knowledge of educational materials (which explain health matters to them).
3. Blacks live on a poorer diet than whites. This exposes them to more fats, more carbohydrates, more salt, more spices, and more carcinogens.
4. Blacks (as a percentage) have the least paying and the most dangerous jobs which expose them often to industrial disease causing agents.
5. The stress of poverty, racism, and bigotry is primarily responsible for the epidemic drug addiction, alcoholism, and AIDS, which are devastating the black community.

According to 1988 statistics, the median survival rate of the black male is 64.9 years. For the white male it is 73.4 years. There is 8.5 years difference in the median survival rate between white and black males. The median survival rate of white female is 78.9 years and for the black female it is 73.0 years. There is a difference of 5.9 in the median survival rate between white and black females. The average life span of black males and black females in this country is 69.2 years. The average life span of white males and white females is 75.6 years. In effect, the white women in this country live 14 years longer than black males. There is 5.5 years difference in the median survival rate between white males and white females. There is also a greater gap of survival rate between the black males and females as opposed to the gap existing between white males and females.

In this book, I outline and explain what a black person can do to improve his or her health and live a longer life.

Introduction

THE INCREASING MORTALITY OF BLACK AMERICANS

THE HEALTH STATUS OF BLACK AMERICANS

The health status of Black Americans is deteriorating and deteriorating fast. According to the latest statistics, the median survival rate for the black male has dropped to 64.9 years in 1991, from 67.7 years in 1987–88. This is one indication that the black community is now seriously threatened and dying sooner. Some major reasons for this situation are outlined and explained in this book, but, the basic reason for this decline is due to a combination of the poor health care that Blacks are receiving and the poor health habits that they presently have. Too much alcohol, smoking, cholesterol, and stress are all leading to the decline of the median survival age. The combination of these conditions is a formula for disaster. If nothing is done to turn this situation around, then the devastation and decline are going to both continue and increase.

REASONS FOR THE HIGH MORTALITY RATE OF BLACK BABIES

Not only is there a decline in the median survival rate of black males, but also the infant mortality rate is increasing. For each one thousand black babies born in the United States, nineteen of them die at birth; but for each one thousand white babies born in the United States, only eight of them die at birth. The reasons for such a high mortality rate are:

1. Poor pre-natal care
2. Alcohol abuse
3. IV drug use
4. Cigarette use
5. Overall poor nutritional care

Alcohol and drug abuse, and cigarette smoking and poor nutrition during pregnancy are all factors which can effect the health of these fetuses negatively. Many of these mothers are teen-agers, and have no money to pay for good prenatal care. Also, they do not like sitting in a hospital Emergency Room for 6–7 hours, or sitting in a clinic for 4–6 hours before they receive attention. And, the clinics are very likely not to be well-equipped or well-staffed. These conditions, combined with problems such as fetal alcohol syndrome, are now taking their toll.

FETAL ALCOHOL SYNDROME

In the case of fetal alcohol syndrome, mothers are consuming alcohol in large quantities while they are pregnant. This leads to birth defects, mental retardation, and a whole host of other problems. The baby is born with a very low Apgar and does not stand a chance to survive. Even if the baby were to survive, the baby is likely to develop brain dysfunction later on in life (a brain that was effected at the time that he/she was in the mother's womb) and will eventually become a burden to society. In the first place, the developing child will not be able to learn in school, and as a result he/she will be unable to become a productive working citizen. Women who are pregnant and use drugs, such as alcohol, cocaine, crack and heroin, are exposing their babies to the development of a multitude of complications and permanent birth defects.

THE STRESS OF RACISM AND ALCOHOLISM IN BLACKS

African-Americans, not only suffering from poverty and diseases, have now an increasingly higher incidence of alcoholism. Because of their suffering and stress, they are trying to ease their pain by cheap intoxication.

And, more African-American women suffer from health problems related to alcoholism than men. This is partly due to the fact that Black women are already suffering from obesity and hypertension. Adding alcoholism to this situation worsens these conditions.

RACISM AND POVERTY IN BLACKS

Racism leads to poverty. Poverty leads to despair and anger. All of this leads to self destructive behaviors such as alcoholism and drug addiction which complicate already poor health habits and drain resources. But, racism also damages the entire human entity (psychologically and physically). It does not just deprive Black American citizens of good jobs, good homes, or good food, but it also indirectly forces many citizens into the streets where they live under subhuman conditions.

ERADICATION OF POVERTY AND ILLITERACY IN BLACKS

It is now the time to eradicate the poverty and illiteracy which leads individuals to negative self-destructive behaviors and bad health. Basically, the African-American community and subsequently the Hispanic community are being decimated systematically by the side effects of racism. One example would be the AIDS epidemic which is presently devastating communities in an excruciating manner. Other diseases that are either killing or crippling Blacks are: hypertension, heart disease, diabetes, eye diseases, arthritis, peptic ulcer disease, tuberculosis, and cancer, and their numerous complications. All these major diseases that are prevalent in the American society affect Blacks at a much higher percentage than their white counterparts.

There is nothing wrong with Black Americans genetically that they should be suffering from these diseases to such a vast extent. It is the poverty, deprivation, and stress that are their malignant root causes.

POOR BLACKS AND CITY HOSPITAL AND CLINICS

Poor Blacks, by and large, receive their medical care from city hospitals, neighborhood clinics and community hospitals. Most of these individuals have no health insurance or depend on Medicaid and Medicare.

In city hospitals, where they have teaching programs, these patients are admitted as ward patients, and they are cared for by doctors in-training under the supervision of attending physicians. These patients, by and large, receive very good medical care. In the voluntary hospital setting, the situation is quite different. If the patient is lucky enough to find a caring, compassionate, and qualified physician, the care is likely to be good, but otherwise it is left to a chance situation as to the quality of the care. In the community clinic setting, the care is often times inadequate, though there are exceptions. Therefore, the vast majority of poor people receive sub-optimal medical care. The reasons are the same reasons why they get sub-optimal treatment in society; unemployment, and lack of sufficient government funding of health care, lack of incentives and, in some instances, the lack of training and knowledge to provide good medical care for these individuals. The poor get poor medical care for the simple reason that they are poor. In a society as rich as ours, this is unconscionable and un-ethical. And, every segment of the American society is being affected, directly or indirectly, by the worsening of our health care system. And, unfortunately the Government has made the delivery of health care in the United States much more difficult.

HEALTH MAINTENANCE ORGANIZATIONS

Health Maintenance Organizations are supposed to provide better health care for less money, which in fact has not happened. The Government has set up a system of DRG's to hold hospitals and doctors accountable for cutting costs of health care delivery. But, this has not happened. It has created a bureaucratic nightmare on the one hand, and on the other hand, it has forced hospitals to administer and to police programs and every day activities that are providing care for patients. Most health professionals could be better used by delivering hands-on care for patients. Billions of dollars are wasted every year to administer bureaucratic medical-watchdog agencies while the health of Blacks and other minorities is deteriorating to catastrophic levels. Monies that could have, and should have, been spent to care for the poor, the disabled, and the elderly, are being unnecessarily wasted.

THE MEDICAID PROGRAM

Systems such as Medicaid were set up to pay for the health care needs of the poor and disabled. But, it is ill conceived that one can justify paying a physician only $9 to $11 per visit to provide care for Blacks, Hispanics, the homeless, the disabled, and the elderly. The poorer the individual, the longer the list of medical problems, and, the more serious medical problems are always present. These individuals need to be treated by the more experienced and competent physicians. But, the medical system does not provide a reasonable medical fee for these physicians to take care of these Medicaid patients. Therefore, the less experienced and less qualified physicians are the ones that are generally taking care of them. All of this is resulting, in part, to the present deteriorating health status of Blacks.

THE HEALTH INSURANCE INDUSTRY

Also, there is a large segment of the American society (numbered in the millions) who have no health insurance at all. When these individuals become seriously ill, they end up in the emergency room and hospitals as indigent patients. The quality of care that is going to be provided for them is being left to chance. They may or may not be lucky enough to find a compassionate, willing, and competent doctor to manage their health problems.

There is another segment who, though they have health insurance, if faced with any serious illness (that lasts more than a few weeks) could cause them financial ruin. The insurance companies are now allowed to pick and choose who they want to insure. Sometimes they terminate somebody's insurance coverage if they suspect that the person's health problems are going to cost them too much money. They do this by raising premiums so high, making it impossible for the payments to be affordable.

SOCIETY AND THE HEALTH CARE SYSTEM FOR THE POOR

Society has the responsibility to provide for the health care needs of its citizens. Black Americans have the right to expect that their health care needs will be provided for. And, this should, and must, include all health care needs, including the cost of medications, etc.

MEDICAL CARE AS A RIGHT

Medical care is a right, not a privilege. So therefore, when going to a doctor, a patient has the right to ask questions. When a doctor agrees to provide medical care, there automatically exists an implied contract. The doctor must do his or her best to provide one with the most competent care possible and must advocate for one's best interest at all times. In addition, the doctor must treat the patient with compassion, understanding, professionalism and the highest ethics. The rights of the patient have to be respected regardless of the patient's socio-economic background. If a certain level of care is being given to one member of a community, and it is not being given to someone else in that community, then something is definitely wrong. Ethically, health care really should know no boundaries. There must be one standard of care for everybody, but unfortunately, this is not our present situation. The poor get the worst care, and the rich get the best care.

PATIENT'S RESPONSIBILITY FOR HIS/HER OWN HEALTH

But also, the patient has a responsibility for his/her own health. One should equip one's self with knowledge so that one knows what are the right questions to ask the physician. This is one of the purposes of this book. In reading this book and becoming aware of the serious medical problems facing Black Americans, the next time a medical problem arises, you will be able to ask the physician intelligent questions.

CORRECTIVE MEASURES TO RESOLVE
THE HEALTH PROBLEMS OF BLACKS

Corrective measures need to be taken to resolve this devastating trend, and our government, society, and African-Americans all need to begin to better their living conditions, and as a result, better their health. Our society should be responsible for providing for the health care needs of its citizens. No American citizen should have to do without good health care or no health care because the Government is failing to carry out its responsibility. Health care translates into life itself, and a Government that would fail in its duties to safeguard the health of its citizens is indeed failing to safeguard the life of its citizens. The United States is the leading country in the world in terms of wealth, weapons, and technology. But, it is low on the list of countries that provide good health care for its citizens. It is disheartening to see the poor health care of the citizens of communities where minorities reside.

THE BLACK MEDIA

Black academicians, scientists, black businessmen and women need to write articles and make radio and television statements and comments dealing with health and economic issues. This needs to be done to reverse this trend of poverty which is resulting in such poor health status and consequently so many early deaths.

Also, the black media (popular black magazines, black newspapers, radio stations and television stations) must begin to bring health information to the black communities. But, this is only the first step to correct the deteriorating trend leading to early deaths of black men, women, and children at such increasing numbers. The black media as a financial entity survives because it is supported by the dollars of black men and women; so it is only fair that it involves itself more than it has in the past, in order to advocate for the betterment of the overall conditions of Blacks. At a time when the economic situation of Blacks has never been worse, and as a result, the overall health of Blacks is deteriorating, the black media must begin to move vigorously to address the issues of drug addiction, alcoholism, AIDS, infant mortality, unemployment and the ever vanishing black family structure. It is, one would think, in the best interest of the black media, to undertake these measures, for this is the only way it can expect to survive. It should begin to encourage Black youngsters to go to school, and stay in school to acquire the necessary skills to ensure a better future for themselves and their families. This is one way in which to proceed to turn around the negative trend that is prevalent in the black community.

BLACK COMMUNITY AND THE ECONOMY

The black community spends an excess of $290 billion per year in order to survive in the American society. Yet, very little, if any, of that money finds its way back to the black community. It is therefore, imperative that a form of business cooperative be organized within the black communities in order to assure economic stability. To do this, there ought to be the development of small business ventures to be owned by black men and women, and there ought to be training programs set up to train individuals from the black community in how to run small businesses. Also, a program for scholarship ought to be set up to aid children to not only become the intellectual professionals, such as: teachers, lawyers, physicians, pharmacists, dentists, accountants, engineers, computer experts, architects, etc. but also to learn trades, such as carpentry, masonry, electrical work, and plumbing. The same goal and commitment that the United States Government used in the Marshall plan ought to be initiated again to bring about such a program.

POVERTY AND THE WEALTH OF THE UNITED STATES OF AMERICA

It is unconscionable for a country as rich as the United States to have such a large segment of its citizens suffering such disproportionate degrees of poverty. What is needed to resolve the problem is better housing, better schooling, better health care, more clinics with more minority physicians, and more hospitals that are well-equipped, well-staffed and well-funded. This would ensure that the African-Americans would have good health care—health care that is delivered by competent, well-trained physicians, nurses and other health care providers. This would decrease the incidence of death and increase the immediate survival of African-Americans. Once this is done, the overall condition of African-Americans in the United States will improve tremendously. If it is not done, we will continue to have an unhealthy segment of society that will continue to suffer unnecessarily.

HOW TO DEAL WITH RACISM AND BIGOTRY

Although racism and bigotry are anger-provoking types of situations, the way to deal with them is not to become angrier in negative ways but rather it is best to engage in doing constructive and positive things. This is the way to overcome the negative impacts of racism and bigotry in a positive manner. Find a way to become employed. Find a way to become better educated and skilled. Find a way to keep one's health as best as one can by learning about health issues and maintaining a reasonable diet. One must have a healthy body and mind to become productive. One has to eradicate misery by work, education, and by staying healthy, and this is the only way that works. This is the formula that is needed in order for the Black community to improve. Racism is not going to go away. It is going to be here until the end of time. As horrible as this sounds, it is one of those hard facts with which one must cope. But, the only way to deal with racism and bigotry is to fight it head on, by becoming successful members of one's community. Even though, when one is successful, one still has to fight racism, at least one is in a position where it can be fought more effectively.

THE ADVANTAGES OF BEING BORN
IN THE UNITED STATES OF AMERICA

Being born an American is in itself a great asset. The United States of America is a country that provides vast opportunities for its citizens. Yet, a large segment of American Blacks and other minorities have failed to take advantage of the opportunities that the United States offers. No doubt, there are obstacles that they must overcome in order to take advantage of these opportunities. But, people have come here with little or no knowledge of the language, and have managed to integrate themselves in the American society and become successful.

THE FORMULA FOR SUCCESS

Again, the formula is very simple. It is hard work and more hard work. It is studying and having a goal, and a desire to achieve and having the motivation to pursue that goal to the end.

THE REASONS FOR WRITING THIS BOOK

In writing this book, I seek to take you through an analysis of the major health problems that face Black Americans. It is my hope that by reading this book that one will find a way to better one's own health. The chapters that follow are my gift to you, my brothers and sisters.

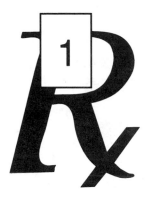

HYPERTENSION AND BLACK PEOPLE

Hypertension and hypertension associated diseases are the leading causes of death for blacks in the United States. Roughly 62 million people in the United States suffer from hypertension, about 43% of these individuals have either poorly controlled or uncontrolled hypertension as reported in *Internal Medicine World Report,* May 1–14, 1991, Vol. 6.

WHAT IS HYPERTENSION?

Hypertension occurs when the blood pressure is elevated beyond the normal range. What is the normal range for blood pressure? The normal range for blood pressure is anywhere from 110 to 139 systolic and from the range of 70 to 88 diastolic.

Some individuals have blood pressures lower than 110, i.e., 100 to 110 systolic and some individuals have a blood pressure between 65–70 systolic. This is still considered normal. Blood pressure therefore, has a range. When is the blood pressure considered elevated? In our system of medicine, blood pressure of 96 diastolic and above is considered elevated; the cut-off point for diastolic is 90. Blood pressure between 70–90 is really accepted as a normal diastolic. A systolic blood pressure of 105–139 is accepted as normal.

Hypertension is associated with the development of arteriosclerotic disease, kidney disease, stroke, and blindness. Heart disease associated with hypertension is the result of hardening of the arteries around the heart,

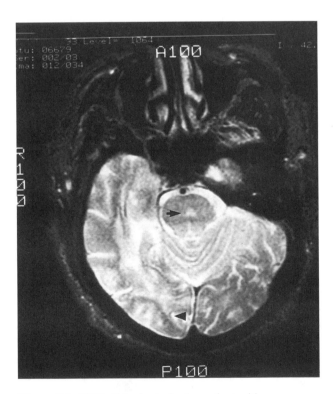

Figure 1.1. MRI of the brain in the patient with hypertension: small infarct in the pon (arrow) and right occipital white matter (arrow head)

referred to as coronary artery disease. Because of the stress that the blood pressure places on the arteries around the heart, the deposition of plaque within the walls of these vessels leads to their clogging. This prevents oxygen from reaching the muscles of the heart in sufficient quantity.

HEART ATTACK

What Is a Heart Attack?

A heart attack occurs when an area of the heart muscle dies as a result of the lack of oxygen to that area. When oxygen fails to reach the heart muscles in sufficient quantity, angina pectoris manifests as chest pain and shortness of breath. Angina pectoris and its many manifestations may be a prodrome to the development of heart attack.

Congestive Heart Failure

High blood pressure (when left untreated, or not treated properly) causes the heart muscle to become enlarged. The muscle has to work harder to pump the heavier load of blood. This will eventually result in congestive heart failure. Congestive heart failure occurs when the heart is no longer able to pump the blood forward. This results in the backing up of fluid in the lungs, in the legs, and sometimes in the abdomen, causing the person to have shortness of breath, and fluid in the lungs. If not treated promptly and appropriately, this will surely result in the death of the individual.

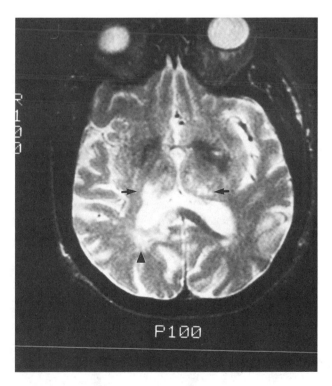

Figure 1.2. MRI of the brain in patient with hypertension: infarction of thalamus (arrows) and right parietal white matter (arrow head)

Kidney Disease

The second problem that high blood pressure can cause is kidney disease. The mechanism through which high blood pressure causes kidney disease is a condition called nephrosclerosis. Nephrosclerosis is the deposition of plaque within the vessels that circulate inside the kidneys (as a result of the high pressure within these vessels) causing them to lose their smoothness. This allows particles to settle within the kidneys. This leads to nephrosclerosis. When this happens, the patient begins to experience an inability to get rid of waste products, resulting ultimately in kidney failure. Kidney failure can be caused by many conditions; however, hypertension is one of the leading causes of kidney failure in blacks.

Once the kidneys fail, (unless the person is treated with dialysis or a kidney transplant) the patient will be unable to get rid of waste products, and will be unable to pass a sufficient amount of urine. The body will accumulate water and a variety of salts and waste products which will lead to death.

Stroke

The third problem associated with hypertension is stroke. Stroke is caused because the pressure within the vessels in the brain is so high, that these vessels lose their integrity. Plaque forms within these walls causing a narrowing of these vessels—thus impeding the flow of blood and oxygen to be delivered to different areas of the brain. This results in a stroke. A stroke may result when a vessel just simply ruptures because the pressure within it is too high. This is called a hemorrhagic stroke.

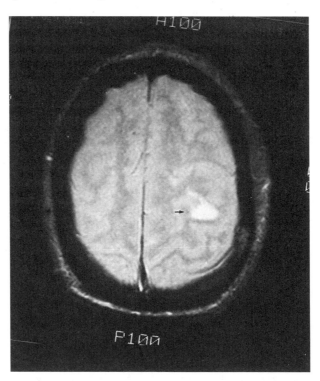

Figure 1.3. MRI of the brain in patient with hypertension: left parietal small infarction. (arrow)

Types of Strokes

There are different types of strokes associated with high blood pressure. Some strokes are the result of damage done to large vessels in the brain; some are the result of a small vessel disease of the brain. Strokes can also result from a disease of the vessels on either side of the neck called carotid arteries. When plaque forms within these vessels in the neck, a pre-stroke condition that often develops is called a transient ischemic attack known as TIA. This means that there is not enough blood being received in the circulation of the brain because of the narrowing of these vessels. It is also important to mention that high cholesterol can also lead to plaque formation which may cause a stroke. Once the stroke develops, death may occur immediately, or the person may become paralyzed in different parts of the body and may require extensive rehabilitation. The possibility of the development of seizures and the many other complications of a stroke may also lead to death.

Hypertension and Blindness

Hypertension is also associated with blindness. Because the vessels within the eye experience tremendous stress from the increased pressure, hemorrhaging within the vessels of the eyes, (if left untreated) can lead to blindness. This will be further discussed in Chapter Eleven, "Eye Diseases".

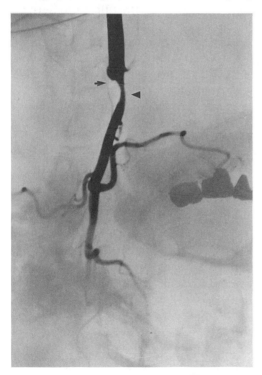

Figure 1.4. Arteriosclerotic disease of carotid arteries in patients with hypertension causing transient ischemic attacks. (pre-stroke syndrome)
Carotid angiogram: occlusion of internal carotid artery at its origin. (arrow); narrowing of proximal internal carotid artery (arrow head).

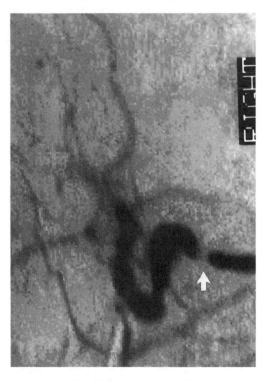

Figure 1.5. Cerebral angiogram 95% occlusion of internal carotid artery in a patient with hypertension. (arrow)

5

THE TREATMENT OF
HYPERTENSION

(1) It is important to know the age of the patient, (2) the weight of the patient, and (3) the work activity of the patient. For instance, blood pressure in the elderly group is treated quite differently from the way that it is treated in the young adult and the middle-aged individual. If the individual is obese and if he or she has a diastolic blood pressure of 90 and a systolic blood pressure of 140, a reduction in weight and a decrease in salt intake will suffice. On the other hand, if the individual has blood pressure of 150 over 94 and if the person is not obese and a non-smoker, then one can set up a diet program to try to reduce salt intake. This procedure might suffice in bringing the blood pressure down. If diet is not sufficient (after two or three examinations of the patient), prescribing a mild water pill would be the first step to bring the blood pressure down to a diastolic below 90 and a systolic below 140.

Special Treatment for Blacks

It is important to note that hypertension in the Caucasian population is quite a different disease from hypertension in the black population. Therefore, the approach to treatment has to be different.

Low Renin Hypertension

There is a system that operates within the kidneys called the renin angiotensin system. This operation leads to salt retention which may result in water retention. This may elevate the blood pressure. Blacks, in general, have low renin in their systems, so they have low renin hypertension.

On the other hand, Caucasians have high renin in their systems, so they have high renin associated hypertension. It is of utmost importance that these facts are kept in mind when one is about to treat a black person for

hypertension. The first medication to be used in treating a black person with hypertension is a diuretic known as a water pill.

Essential Hypertension

About ninety-eight percent of blacks who are hypertensive are hypertensive because they have essential hypertension. Essential hypertension is basically the type of hypertension that has its roots in the genetic transmission of the disease from the fore-parents of blacks. The kidneys of black individuals are unable to get rid of salt in sufficient amounts because of a genetic abnormality.

Some three hundred years ago, in Africa, it was necessary for Blacks to develop a way in which to prevent salt wastage from the kidneys in an attempt to prevent the loss of water from the body, thereby preventing dehydration. When working on the farms, far away from easy access to water, where the sun is very hot, and a great deal of sweating takes place, much salt is lost with the sweat, taking water with it. Were it not for this mechanism, whereby the kidney is able to re-absorb salt through its tubules, dehydration, leading to collapse of the intravascular system, leading to death, would have been the mechanism of dying of these individuals. Not only was this the case for Blacks, long ago in Africa, but also now in the tropical countries. It is a common practice in the tropics to carry water in calabashes to the farm to drink sparingly, to last from 7 A.M. until 6 P.M. So, the use of water is tightly controlled, because frequently these individuals are working far away from a source of drinking water. This survival gene helped keep the black slaves alive during the long journey from Africa to the Americas, and helped further in their survival while working in the cotton fields, and the sugar cane fields in the hot sun. The author C. L. R. James describes in his book, *The Black Jacobins*, the horrible

6

conditions in which Blacks were brought from Africa to the new world, and how these conditions clearly exposed them to hunger, thirst, and diseases of all types. So, what was then evolved as a survival gene in the old world, had now become a detrimental gene leading to the disease "essential hypertension" in the new world, and all its multitude of complications.

Hypersympathetic Hypertension

Also, there is a form of hypertension seen in both black and white in the 30–55 years range, whose blood pressure fluctuates because of stress. This is called hypersympathetic hypertension, which means that the blood pressure is associated with an overactive nervous system. These individuals respond very well to small doses of Beta Blockers. These shut off, to some extent, the sympathetic flow which brings the blood pressure down. In these subgroups of patients, it is inappropriate to treat them with a diuretic (water pill). The reason for the elevation of blood pressure in these individuals (both Caucasian and non-Caucasian) is not due to salt retention. It is important to stress that some Caucasians have salt retention associated hypertension due to an entirely different mechanism requiring treatment with a diuretic (water pill) to control their blood pressure.

The Need for Diuretics

Therefore, unless one treats a black person with a water pill as part of the medication or as part of a group of medication, the blood pressure of the black person will not respond. Even if the blood pressure responds initially, on large doses of ACE inhibitors, beta blockers, or calcium channel blockers, within a matter of weeks, the blood pressure will level off and again will start to rise. It is therefore inaccurate to treat blacks with monotherapy (only one medication) of

anything other than a diuretic (water pill). However, there are blacks whose blood pressure is so high at presentation that to start treatment with a diuretic alone is not sufficient. In this case, any number of groups of medication mentioned above can be used to start treatment. In the treatment of hypertension of a black person it is essential to include a water pill to eliminate the salt. Once the salt is eliminated, then retention is eliminated and blood pressure is under control. Sometimes, however, it takes three medications to control the blood pressure, but these should not be given in massive doses.

The Need for Beta Blockers

There is a small percentage of blacks and non-blacks who are hypertensive because of renovascular disease which is an obstruction in the circulation of the kidney. This results in blockage causing elevation of renin. These individuals require beta blockers because their renin is high. However, this is a very rare disease, but it may be detected very easily through physical examination. One should listen to the flanks of the patient on both sides of the abdomen and try to hear an abnormal sound which is associated with this condition. If one does not detect this abnormality, then an IVP (a test of the kidney called pyelogram) (intravenous) will detect this abnormality.

Renovascular hypertension is the result of either atherosclerosis roughly 60% of the time or fibromuscular dysplasia about 40% of the time. This condition is associated with the elevation of a substance produced by the kidney name Renin. Renin mediates the conversion of Angiotensinogen to Angiotensin I; this then works upon a convertin enzyme changing into a substance called Angiotensin II which causes vasal constriction of vessels within the kidney. This process then leads to the production of a substance called Aldosterone which then causes sodium to be reabsorbed in the kidney tubules leading to increased intravascular volume raising blood pressure. In this setting, a beta blocker is most appropriate to prevent the elevation of renin, via the blockage of beta receptors that are found within the kidney. This then is the mechanism whereby beta blockers work to reduce hypertension in the high renin setting.

Pheochromocytoma

There is also a condition called pheochromocytoma which is a tumor involving the adrenal gland that is situated on either side of the kidneys. This condition is associated with the production of catecholamine which causes the blood pressure to rise. Catecholamine belong to the family of substances that are secreted by the body called adrenalin. However, the incidence of pheochromocytoma and renovascular hypertension is so rare, that it is not necessary to involve a patient with hypertension, in an extensive evaluation looking for these conditions prior to a treatment trial for the more usual type of hypertension.

TESTING AND EVALUATION OF HYPERTENSION

A physical examination, a urinalysis, a complete blood count, a renal profile, (blood test for the kidney), blood sugar, chest x-ray and an EKG are all one needs in order to have an initial overview of the status of the patient's hypertension and to begin treatment. (1) The EKG is used to see if the patient has had cardiac damage; (2) the chest x-ray is used to see if the heart has been enlarged; (3) the urinalysis is used to see if the patient has protein, red cells, and other materials in the sediment of the urine. If present, these may indicate that the kidney has been damaged.

The blood test for the kidney function is also essential to see how much damage has been done to the kidneys. A complete blood count is needed because anemia is associated with kidney disease resulting from high blood pressure.

Ninety percent of the information obtained from these basic tests is all that one needs to have a general overview of the patient's health so that treatment can be started. When adequate medication and good compliance by the patient fails to control the blood pressure, one should begin to think of other things such as renovascular and pheochromocytoma as underlying causes of the patient's hypertension. However, the evaluation that is involved to search for these conditions is very expensive and should only be performed if necessary. However, the recommended procedures are inexpensive and can be performed in a doctor's office.

HYPERTENSION AND DIET

Diet adds to the problem of blacks with hypertension. A diet which is too salty, too greasy, and too spicy, (so-called soul food), is very harmful to one's health. Because of the high salt content of this type of diet, blood pressure rises. As mentioned before, the high salt intake leads to water retention which leads to high blood pressure. Also, excess water leads to obesity which also causes the pressure to rise. Obesity also is associated with hypertension which will be discussed in the next chapter.

Since the black person's kidney is unable to get rid of the necessary amount of salt as part of a genetic defect, the problem is two-fold: (1) the kidney cannot get rid of salt appropriately, and (2) the diet is too rich in salt. The total of all these factors hastens the process of hypertension. This may lead to cardiac disease and other associated complications of hypertension which may lead to an early death. Most blacks eat this type of diet because of poverty. Blacks buy the cheapest food with the most fats in it. Therefore, they put a high amount of seasoning and salt in it to make it palatable. Also, "junk foods" are loaded with cholesterol and salt. If blacks continue to eat this diet constantly, they are guaranteeing the development of poor health.

Change in Diet to Decrease Hypertension

What can the black person do to decrease the incidence of high blood pressure that may result in stroke, heart disease, kidney failure and blindness? They need to change their dietary habits to foods containing less salt, less fat, and less carbohydrates, thereby lowering cholesterol. By doing so, the person is decreasing the possibility of hypertension and its devastating complications. Therefore, if a black person is being treated by a doctor for hypertension, the doctor should be prescribing him/her a diuretic. If a water pill is not prescribed, there may be a reason for it. Sometimes, uremia due to kidney failure is present, therefore a diuretic may not be appropriate at this point. In people aged 60 and above taking the water pill, one must have a potassium replacement. Eating a banana or drinking orange juice may not be enough. In the younger-age group or middle-aged group the need for potassium replacement is much less. Water pills (diuretics) in the elderly have to be used very carefully. These individuals lose potassium more quickly and they are less likely to eat a proper diet. Therefore, it is important to carefully monitor the electrolytes and the kidney function. Regardless of the age group of the individual, when taking large doses of a diuretic, potassium replacement is always necessary.

Potassium and Renal Failure

However, for individuals with renal failure, potassium intake can be very dangerous. When one has renal failure, taking potassium should only be done under the strictest medical supervision. Once the kidney has failed; it is not able to excrete potassium in the urine. This remaining potassium can cause severe cardiac complications lead-

ing to death. The reverse is also dangerous. For example, low serum potassium can lead to irregularities of the heart, cramping of the legs, weakness, and can lead to death. It is important to keep these issues in mind. If seeing a physician, ask questions. If one is not satisfied with the answers, look around for other health advisors, especially in the case of hypertension.

HYPERTENSION AND THE ELDERLY

Hypertension in the elderly must be handled differently. In the elderly, the systolic blood pressure has a tendency to be higher. It is not always necessary to bring the systolic blood pressure down. The reason for this is because the muscles in the elderly have lost their tone. Therefore, they have wide pulse pressure which means that the difference between the systolic blood pressure and the diastolic blood pressure becomes wider. Higher systolic blood pressure is needed so that the elderly person can perfuse their brain more appropriately.

Treatment in the Elderly

In treating the elderly, carefully use smaller doses of medication than usual. If the systolic blood pressure is in the range of 150, it should be left alone. If the systolic blood pressure drops to the range of normal, (for a young person), it may cause the elderly person to have a stroke. This decreasing of the blood pressure prevents the elderly person from having enough pressure to perfuse the brain. They need a higher pressure because the vessels in the brain become narrower due to arteriosclerotic disease. A blood pressure in the range of 110 systolic may be too low; therefore, keep it in the range of 140–150. Do not add too much medication when treating an elderly person. Slowly add one medication, a small dose, and then wait a week. If readjustment is necessary, add a smaller dose to the medication. Dropping the blood pressure too low may cause a fatality.

Chronic Renal Problems in the Elderly

Renal problems in the elderly may be caused because they are not drinking enough fluids. Do not prescribe water pills if dehydration is detected. Diuretics will decrease the intravascular system which may collapse, causing strokes, heart attacks, and other complications. The doctor has to be very careful with the treatment of blood pressure in the elderly patient. If not, it will cause more harm than good. One of the rules in treating blood pressure in the elderly is to take it in both arms because the blood pressure may be normal in one arm, but very high in the other. The patient may have a plaque causing obstruction in the arteries in one arm, resulting in a low blood pressure. However, the blood pressure in an uninvolved arm may have a very high blood pressure. So, to repeat, it is very important to take the blood pressure in both arms.

Blood Pressure and the Elderly

Also, taking blood pressure in the elderly should be done lying, sitting, and standing. If the elderly person is unable to stand, take the blood pressure lying and sitting. When a patient lies down, the blood pressure, for example, may be 180/70, but, if the same elderly person sits up for about five minutes, it may be 150/70 if taken again. This is perfectly acceptable for an elderly person. If standing up and one waits another five minutes, the blood pressure may be 130/60. If one were to treat this elderly patient when lying down and the blood pressure was 180/70, that doctor could cause a catastrophe.

If an elderly person talks about being dizzy, think about other things including: transient ischemic attacks, cardiac arrhythmias, and heart blocks that cause dizziness. Although this may signify some kind of pre-stroke syndrome, the possibility of orthostatic hypotension may also be present and should be carefully diagnosed.

DIURETICS AND DIABETES

Recently, the effect of diuretics on diabetes and on cholesterol have been brought into the forefront. The fact is that diuretics cannot cause diabetes. If diuretics (water pills) are taken and blood sugar rises, the patient may have been diabetic to begin with. The mechanism through which diuretics cause hyperglycemia, namely high blood sugar, is the tendency for one to lose potassium with the urine as an effect of the diuretics. The low potassium causes the receptors found in the Beta cells to be resistant to the effect of secreting insulin. This mechanism causes the blood sugar to rise. If this happens, the person must have underlying dormant sub-clinical diabetes mellitus, or is already a known diabetic causing blood sugar to rise because of hypokalemia (low potassium). If hypokalemia is corrected or prevented, then a blood sugar will not rise because of the effect of the water pill. Potassium replacement should be taken to prevent hypokalemia. When this is done there will be no effect on the blood sugar because the diuretic's effects would have been negated. As stated before, diuretics do not cause diabetes and the slight effect on cholesterol is meaningless. The increase of cholesterol that occurs is a very minuscule part of hypercholesterolemia, or as a result of treating high blood pressure with a diuretic (water pill).

THE NEED FOR BETTER HEALTH CARE FOR THE BLACK COMMUNITY

Health conditions of Blacks in this country are much worse than in some third world countries. This is a shameful situation in the United States of America, (the richest country in the world). It has a subgroup of its citizens, namely blacks, dying unnecessary deaths because of a lack of doctors and better clinics. There exists a poor people's health care crisis. Blacks need to know what to do to try to better their health. The health care system has not provided this information for them. If it had, then the crisis that exists now would never have occurred. Two-thirds of the deaths in the black community are due to poor health care delivery. In fact, the health situation involving two-thirds of the sub-groups of blacks in this country is worse than the health care in some Third World countries. It is grossly sinful that American citizens should be receiving such inadequate outrageous medical care as the result of ignorance, racism, and bigotry. Most blacks in this country receive their medical care from poorly staffed clinics where the patients don't challenge this type of inadequate medical care. To resolve this crisis, better trained and qualified doctors, better trained nurses, more equipment, and more medication to stock the clinics are needed.

In addition, the black community must demand from the elected officials that the necessary funding is provided to carry out better health care. Elected black officials ought to question what they should be doing to try to correct this issue. The Health and Human Services Administration, along with other government agencies responsible for funding the health care system in this country, must correct the disastrous health problems that exist in the black community.

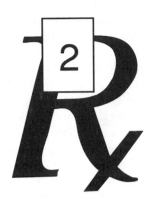

DIET, OBESITY AND HIGH CHOLESTEROL

CHAPTER OUTLINE

OVERVIEW:
DIET, HEART DISEASE, AND STRESS

Diet is one of the main reasons why the death rate of Black Americans is higher than the death rate of White Americans.

The diet of White Americans seems to be better controlled with less fat, less red meat, more polyunsaturated oil and more exercise; while, as previously mentioned, the diet of the black population is saturated with fat, red meat, and too much salt. Whether one believes it or not, in general, Black Americans tend to exercise less than White Americans. This results in a higher incidence of heart disease, namely atherosclerotic heart disease, which leads to heart attack and death. This disease has been decreasing within the last several years in the white population, but it has been increasing at an alarming rate in the black population, primarily due to an unhealthy diet.

The overall living conditions of Blacks is alarmingly worse than that of the white because Blacks are poorer, less educated, have the worst jobs, and more stress (the stress of racism and poverty). All of these combined lead to the worsening death rate in the black population.

DIET

Diet is very important regardless of the fact that one is poor. If one has the know-how, one can intermix one's food in such a way as to better the diet. The poor diet leads to obesity and stomach problems of different sorts. It also leads to hypertension, which in turn leads to multiple complications.

If Blacks were to eat more vegetables, more fruits, less fat, less red meat, this would improve a great deal the overall situation of the state of black health in this country. Fish is very good. Chicken is very good. If possible, removing the skin of the chicken to remove the excess fat is helpful. Meat, such as veal, is very good. But, red meat such as beef and pork, though they may have tremendous protein value, have too much fat. The fat that is found in red meat is saturated fat which is pure cholesterol and triglyceride. These fats will ultimately cause an increase in the lipid substances in the blood leading to deposition in the vessels which in turn causes atherosclerotic heart disease. Too much bread, too much sugar, and other types of carbohydrates are also bad because the liver transforms them into triglycerides, which is a form of fat that one wants to avoid to prevent obesity. High cholesterol and high triglyceride can result in atherosclerotic heart disease and early death.

OBESITY

Obesity is a health problem for the black community because it is associated with high triglycerides; Diabetes Mellitus, heart disease, and hypertension.

Black women have a tendency to become more obese than white women. Obesity, (ruling out hypothyroidism and other associated endocrine abnormalities), is a genetic disease. The gene is transmitted, from parents to offspring. This gene promotes low metabolism. Low metabolism means that ingested carbohydrates have difficulty burning. Therefore, they are transformed into fat. This fat remains in the body which leads to obesity and all its complications.

Decreased Carbohydrates

What can one do to deal with obesity? First of all, one has to understand that this is a lifelong problem. Any quick weight losing diet does not remain effective due to prior habits, and the fact that it is a genetic disease. One has to begin a program of exercise and decreased carbohydrate ingestion. One has to decrease carbohydrate intake and exercise in order to increase metabolism and burn off the excess carbohydrate.

Recommended Diet

Select a diet that is high in protein and low in carbohydrates. Protein is needed because every day one breaks down protein and more is needed to make new amino acid to replace the protein that has been lost. Ingestion of protein, no matter the amount, will not cause weight gain. One can eat all the food one wants, and all the protein one wants without weight gain. Therefore, if a diet is organized in such a way so that it includes plenty of vegetables, fruits and protein, one will lose weight slowly. The natural carbohydrates that are ingested from fruits is more than enough carbohydrate for sustenance. Especially, if one's liver is full of stored carbohydrate due to an inability to burn it, a condition that is associated with low metabolism, as stated above.

Example of a low carbohydrate, high protein and low fat diet is 800 calories or 100 grams of carbohydrate, 100–150 grams of protein, and 25–35 grams of fat per day.

OBESITY AND DIABETES

Also, there is a significant association between Diabetes Mellitus, Type II (a genetically transmitted form of diabetes) which is associated with obesity. The reason is that the fat cells become resistant to the effects of insulin. The insulin cannot penetrate the fat cells as it would in a normal person. That is one of the mechanisms of insulin resistance in people who are obese. As a result, if one were fated, as it were, to be diabetic genetically, then that situation becomes more likely. If one is obese, diabetic, and is taking medication for the diabetes, unless one loses weight, it will be almost impossible to be treated with either an oral agent, a pill, or with insulin. The more insulin one receives when obese, the more obese one may become. Insulin is an anabolic agent. It increases the appetite. One should not increase the insulin, but rather lose weight. If one loses weight, the need for insulin lessens. As a matter of fact, a non-insulin requiring diabetic may lose weight on a diet that is well organized. This may be sufficient to control the blood sugar. Once weight is lost, the fat cells will become less resistant to insulin. Native insulin that is still left in the pancreas will now begin to secrete in order to control the blood sugar adequately. This also may decrease any necessitating of medication. A low carbohydrate diet is really the saving future for the obese diabetic.

OBESITY AS A MEDICAL PROBLEM

Obesity is a medical problem, not just a cosmetic one. Recently, several reports have shown that obesity is associated with coronary artery disease. According to these reports, truncal obesity (obesity around the trunk of the body) is associated with coronary artery disease. The obese person tends to secrete more insulin. Because of the natural resistance of insulin that exists in obesity, the body seems to want more and more insulin to break down a given amount of blood sugar. As the result of that, the insulin seems to be one of the substances that are associated with the formation of plaques within coronary arteries which can lead to coronary artery disease, myocardial infarction, and death. As important as it is to look good, it is just as important to lose weight for health purposes. Obesity is a medical problem, and unless handled carefully and properly, it will lead to early death.

HIGH CHOLESTEROL

High Cholesterol is a term that means, in the generic sense, hyperlipidemia. Hyperlipidemia is associated with both high cholesterol and high triglycerides, and in some instances, a combination of both high cholesterol and high triglycerides. The liver either makes them or biosynthesizes them. They are naturally needed for the integrity of blood vessels. Cholesterol is needed as a building block, a skeletal block needed to form natural hormones. But, there are genetic conditions that cause the liver to make more of these substances. As mentioned, this genetic abnormality is called hyperlipidemia. Also, there are some conditions of hyperlipidemia which prevent some lipid substances from being broken down by the liver. These are absorbed by the bile, and then are passed into the bowel. From there they are excreted with the stool.

Hyperlipidemia

In diagnosing hyperlipidemia, one must keep in mind that there are five types. They are:

Type 1 which is associated with chylomicron, which leads to the formation of high triglycerides.

Type 2A which is associated with low density lipoprotein, LDL. This is a result of high cholesterol.

Type 2B which is associated with both LDL and VLDL (low density lipoprotein and very low density lipoprotein), which leads to both high cholesterol and high triglycerides.

Type 3 which is associated with both high cholesterol and high triglyceride in greater degrees.

Type 4 which is associated with high very low density lipoprotein VLDL and high triglyceride VLDL.

Type 5 which is associated with a high level of VLDL (very low density lipoprotein) and chylomicron. This results in high triglycerides and high cholesterol.

DIFFERENT TYPES OF CHOLESTEROL

Also, there are different types of cholesterol. The most important type is the high density lipoprotein (HDL). The HDL is important because it takes the bad cholesterol out of the blood, and brings it back into the liver, where it can be broken down into bile acids and carried into the bile. Then, this bad cholesterol passes into the colon where it mixes with the stool and is excreted.

If one has high cholesterol, one should try to decrease the total cholesterol while attempting to increase the HDL. If the HDL is increased to 55 mg/dl. or greater, the risk of coronary artery disease decreases. However, if the HDL is low, (less than 55 mg/dl.) and the LDL and the cholesterol are still remaining high, then the chances of having early coronary artery disease and/or a heart attack as early as the age of 30 increases.

Black women have a tendency to be obese, hypertensive, and have higher cholesterol. The advantage that women are supposed to have over men below age 50 has been negated in black women. White women, on the other hand, have less incidence of hypertension, less incidence of early coronary artery disease, because of lower levels of cholesterol.

Black males have higher incidences of hypertension, obesity and higher cholesterol than the white male. Diet plays a big role. Hypercholesterolemia, namely high cholesterol, is not only associated with genetically transmitted hyperlipidemia, but also other conditions associated with high cholesterol, such as alcoholism, diabetes Mellitus, hypothyroidism, uremia, biliary cirrhosis, and many others.

The black man lives under constant stress because of racism, bigotry, and poverty. Therefore, it is not difficult to see why the level of cholesterol in Blacks is much higher than white males. Emotional stress has been associated with increased secretion of very low density lipoprotein and also decreased breakdown of very low density lipoprotein. Also, the overall incidence of coronary artery disease and myocardial infarction has decreased in the white population while it is increasing at an alarming rate in the black population due to worsening living conditions.

DECREASING CHOLESTEROL

One should eat a diet that has ample fruits, vegetables, polyunsaturated fat such as corn oil, vegetable oil, a lot of fish, chicken without the skin and turkey. Avoid red meat, milk, cheese, shellfish, butter, avocado and coconut. Avoid red meat such as pork and beef in particular. It is not difficult to see why there is such a high incidence of coronary artery disease, myocardial infarction, and death in the black population. Because the black population is poorer, it is not able to buy foods that are less fatty. Therefore, Blacks eat what they can afford. A diet that is poorly conceived and poorly organized. Even when black people achieve middle-class American status, they tend to carry the same old, poor eating habits—even when they can afford better food. Diet is cultural. No matter who we are, what we are, what position is attained in life, one eats the food that one is raised on. Consequently, a black family may move into the best neighborhood and still adheres to a poor diet. When they prepare their meals at home, most go right back to the grits and sausages, bacon and eggs, hogs and pigtails, and collard greens, rich foods that are deadly.

THE USE OF MEDICATIONS TO LOWER CHOLESTEROL

The best medication available for lowering cholesterol is Lovastatin, (Mevacor). It has the least side effects, and it is the most effective. It works as a direct inhibitor of an enzyme (HMGCOA Reductase) which is needed for cholesterol synthesis in the liver. So, Mevacor prevents the production of cholesterol by the liver and decreases its level in the blood. The dosage of the medication is to be left to the physician based on the degree of hypercholesterolemia in the patient. But, this medication may have some minor gastrointestinal side effects. Also, anyone taking this medication is advised to have an eye examination prior to taking the medication, and then be re-examined a couple of times a year. The medication can also cause some cramping of the legs. This may lead to some muscle breakdown that can cause high potassium. But, these side effects are not seen frequently, and this is the best medication to lower cholesterol. Of course, the first step should be a change in diet, and one should resort to medication when diet fails.

If the cholesterol is high, (300 mg/dl. or greater), it is going to be very difficult to bring this cholesterol down to a reasonable level of 200 mg/dl. or lower without intervention with medication. Unfortunately, some of these medications are quite expensive.

Another medication that may lower cholesterol is Cholestyramine. This traps the bile acid, (preventing it from going back into the liver), and diverts it back into the bile, and then into the colon where it excretes with the stool. But, it has significant side effects. It causes constipation, bloating, and cramping.

Another cholesterol lowering medication that may be prescribed in Niacin. Again, this medication can cause flushing and headaches. It has to be taken in large doses, and it is not the most effective of the medications for lowering cholesterol.

Presently, the best medication to lower the triglyceride is Lopid. High triglyceride is known to be associated with heart disease. When it is found elevated along with the cholesterol, it increases the possibility of atherosclerotic heart disease even more.

Lopid can cause some liver function test abnormality and some bloating and cramping in the stomach, but these are reasonably tolerable side effects. Anyone who takes Lopid and Lovastatin is advised to have the liver function tests evaluated every six weeks or so. If the liver function tests are found to be very abnormal, the medication has to be stopped or readjusted downwards.

HIGH TRIGLYCERIDES

When triglyceride elevation occurs, it is necessary to institute a low carbohydrate diet. Because the liver converts carbohydrates into triglycerides, the lowering of triglyceride to any degree depends on a low carbohydrate diet (anywhere from 1200 calories to 1500 calories). If the triglyceride is high, this has to be dealt with individually involving the patient and the doctor and the circumstances.

THE NEED FOR EXERCISE

Exercise is known to increase the HDL, and if one increases one's HDL, one is in the right direction for the prevention of coronary artery disease. Therefore, exercise is paramount. Poorer Blacks, because the menial jobs that most of them have, get up early to go to work, work later and longer hours, and don't have the strength, the capability, or the facilities to exercise. Most poor black women do menial work. When they come home, they have to deal with children and other associated problems, and also do not have time to exercise. The middle-class Blacks and the upper-middle-class Blacks who are able to exercise and eat a better diet, are going to be healthier and live longer. There is no genetic predisposition that Blacks should have worse cases of coronary artery disease than whites. It is only a question of lifestyle. If one is poor and unable to eat a good diet and exercise, (regardless of your race), then one is at a higher risk to develop coronary artery disease. But, because Blacks are poorer, using the Harlem Community in New York City for example, thirty to thirty-five percent of the deaths that take place in that community are associated with alcoholism, drugs, and AIDS. But, sixty to sixty-five percent are really associated with conditions such as cancer, coronary heart disease, heart attacks, high blood pressure, and stroke. Cirrhosis of the liver is also increased another thirty to thirty-five percent.

DIET, OBESITY, HEART DISEASE, AND SMOKING

If one has poor diet, hyperlipidemia, which is high cholesterol, high triglyceride or a combination of both, that is known as a risk factor for heart disease and early death. Hypertension is a risk factor for heart disease. Obesity is a risk factor for heart disease. Cigarette smoking is an important factor as well. Cigarettes contain substances such as nicotine and nicotine is associated with increased incidence of heart disease. The incidence of smoking, alcoholism, hypertension and high cholesterol in Blacks as stated above, is very high. Therefore, the combination of the above problems explains the disastrous nature of the poor health of the black community as it relates to heart disease and other assorted deadly diseases.

Example of an excellent diet for weight reduction and the maintenance of good health is "The Third World Tropical Weight Control Diet and Health Maintenance Program":

| **Table 3.1** Foods to Avoid | **Table 3.2.** Food to Eat |
No	Yes
Sugar	Seltzer or Water
Beer	All Fruits
Alcohol	All Vegetables
Wine	Natural Fruit Juice
Rice	Egg Whites
Potatoes	Chicken (Broiled)
Red Meat	Fish (Broiled)
Pork	Veal (Broiled)
Starch of Any Kind	Only Vegetable Oil
Cheese	Salad with Oil and Vinegar Only
Avocado	Tuna
Bread	Turkey
Coconut	4 Gram Sodium
Preservatives	1,000 Calorie Diet
No Added Salt	100–150 Gram Proteins
Oysters	100 Gram Carbohydrates or 800 Calories
Lobsters	30 Grams Fat (Polyunsaturated Oil)
Shrimp	Supplementary Vitamins
Crabs	Trace Elements and Minerals
Egg Yolks	To Be Prescribed by Physicians
Sausage	Daily Exercise
Bacon	Buy Small Scale to Weigh Foods

Complete medical evaluations is recommended prior to starting this diet and the exercise program and it is recommended that continuous medical supervision be done to ensure the maintenance of good health. A breakdown of this diet is purposefully not outlined.

This diet is the sole property of Valiere Alcena, M.D., F.A.C.P.

All rights reserved and no part of this diet should be copied in any form without expressed written permission from Valiere Alcena, M.D., F.A.C.P.

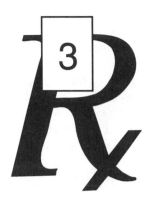

DIABETES MELLITUS
AND
ITS COMPLICATIONS

CHAPTER OUTLINE

DIABETES AND ITS PROBLEMS

Diabetes is a very serious disease that affects many organs in the body. Diabetes can cause blindness. Diabetes Mellitus is also associated with coronary disease. It is associated with kidney disease resulting in renal failure leading to chronic dialysis. Diabetes Mellitus is also associated with generalized arteriosclerosis resulting in vascular disease of a severe nature that can lead to amputation of a limb, namely the foot or the leg. Diabetes Mellitus is also associated with sexual impotence in males. Diabetes Mellitus is also associated with severe peripheral neuropathy that can be very debilitating in some individuals resulting in chronic pain and ulcer, with marked disability.

DIABETES TYPE II

There are two types of Diabetes Mellitus. One type is called Type I, or Juvenile Diabetes, which is associated with a daily insulin requirement. The other type is called Type II, or Adult Onset Diabetes.

The type I diabetes has no known pathophysiological agent responsible for its cause. It is believed that it could be due to a virus attacking the pancreas resulting in destruction of the beta cell of the pancreas. Or, it could be due to some form of autoimmune phenomena resulting in the pancreatic beta cell reacting against itself.

An autoimmune phenomena is a condition in which the body reacts against itself resulting in the destruction of cellular elements.

On the other hand, the Type II Diabetes Mellitus is a genetically transmitted disease whereby an individual develops the inability to break down his/her blood sugar. This is an inability to metabolize the sugar into its component part which leads to elevation of the blood sugar.

Juvenile Diabetes can start at infancy, but, Adult Onset Diabetes usually begins in the mid-thirties. However, any time (age 30–35 onward) an individual might develop diabetes if they have a genetic predisposition. But, there are exceptions to these rules. Juvenile Diabetes behaves as Adult Onset Diabetes, and a small percentage of Adult Onset Diabetes behaves as Juvenile Diabetes. So, (except for the few exceptions), one can readily make the distinction between Juvenile Diabetes and Adult Onset Diabetes clinically.

DIABETES AND THE PANCREAS

The pancreas, (an organ that is found on the left side of the abdomen), has multiple functions. Among its functions is the production of insulin. When an individual eats carbohydrates of different types, insulin is secreted in response to the ingestion of carbohydrates. Natively made carbohydrates in the biochemistry of the body cause secretions of insulin to break down the carbohydrates, known as blood sugar.

So, if the pancreas is damaged, this leads to chronic pancreatitis, which is a third way of becoming diabetic. This type of diabetes has nothing to do with genetics. It is just a destruction of the pancreas that results in the lack of insulin production that causes the blood sugar to rise, resulting in Diabetes Mellitus as well as a variety of other very severe conditions such as diarrhea, associated with a chronic pancreatitis. Because the pancreas secretes the substances that are needed for one to digest fat, if one has no functioning pancreas, fats cannot be digested and this can lead to chronic diarrheal conditions.

DIABETES AND ARTERIOSCLEROSIS

The pathophysiology through which diabetes causes these problems is generalized arteriosclerosis. This results in the hardening of the vessels which results in a lack of blood flow to these different organs which cause generalized problems. There is also generalized damage that occurs to the peripheral nerves which results also in problems. In the eye, for instance, there are several degrees of diabetic retinopathy that, if left untreated, can result in blindness. As for the heart, Diabetes Mellitus is a risk factor for arteriosclerotic heart disease because it causes vascular abnormalities with the formation of plaque. This leads to the obstruction of the blood flow to coronary arteries which leads to coronary artery heart disease. In the kidneys, Diabetes Mellitus can cause diabetic nephropathy which is caused by the deposition of plaque and hardening of the circulatory vessels in the kidney. This generally results in kidney failure. Also, people inflicted with Diabetes Mellitus Type II have a high incidence of chronic renal failure.

The reason why the individuals who have Diabetes Mellitus are predisposed to developing poor circulation, (leading to peripheral vascular disease), is because of the hardening of the arteries and other vessels that are responsible for blood flow. This leads to stasis and lack of blood flow when the individual sustains other trauma to the lower limbs. This develops into poor perfusion of the limbs because of the inability of the blood to carry oxygen to that area. This results in complications that can lead to loss of a foot or limb. A loss of different toes can result in gangrene or other type of infection. It is difficult to treat diabetic foot ulcers or leg ulcers. The vessels are damaged and blood is not feeding the area, so proper healing can't take place.

DETERMINING THE SYMPTOMS OF DIABETES

The presence of diabetes may be detected by routine blood chemistries. Especially when the patient has fasted the night before and the blood sugar is found to be elevated. An elevated blood sugar is a blood sugar of one hundred and thirty to one hundred and fifty. A normal blood sugar in most laboratories is up to one hundred and twenty.

If the blood sugar is found to be elevated in an adult who has a family history of diabetes, then the patient may be diabetic. If the fasting blood sugar is elevated, then a glucose tolerance test is probably not needed.

Other ways for individuals to suspect that they are diabetic are when they begin to feel very thirsty and pass urine very frequently. If they are passing urine very frequently, they may lose a lot of weight and feel tired with general malaise, (chronic fatigue). [These are all signs of the possibility that a person may be diabetic.] In a man, the first sign that diabetes may be developing is that he suddenly becomes impotent (an inability to have an erection or other type of sexual dysfunction). Or in a woman, these may be chronic recurrent vaginal infection, which also may be the first sign of diabetes since the urine contains sugar in a high level, it is a good medium for fungus to grow. As a result, the general area of the vagina is going to grow fungus which cause vaginitis.

In the male, there may be an infection in the foreskin of the glans penis called Balanitis. The infection occurs because the urine contains a high level of sugar which allows for fungus to grow in the foreskin of the penis resulting in infection.

Also, there may be a frequent rash in the groin (both in men and women) because of the possibility of fungal dermatitis associated with diabetes. The frequent passing of urine, (polyuria and polydipsia), (the desire to drink a lot of water), is because a high blood sugar constitutes a type of diuretic. The person is forced to drink a lot of water to replace the water that is being lost in the urine. If allowed to go untreated, the person may reach a stage of Diabetic Mellitus called Diabetic Ketoacidosis. This can lead to coma, and if left untreated can lead to death. Therefore it is very, very important to go to the physician and get examined if experiencing these symptoms.

JUVENILE DIABETES

The presentation of Juvenile Diabetes is somewhat similar. If the chid is found to be not thriving, and has a poor attention span, and generally looks sick, then this child should be evaluated by a pediatrician and blood tests ought to be done quickly to determine what could be wrong with the child.

Diabetic Ketoacidosis

Often one finds out that the chid is diabetic. If the parents wait too long, sometimes the child winds up in an emergency room in a coma as the result of Diabetic Ketoacidosis. This is a tragic situation for it can lead to the death of the child if not treated properly.

Non-Ketotic Hyperosmolar

Another form of diabetes that can be lethal (if not recognized and treated properly) is non-ketotic hyperosmolar state. This is when the blood sugar is very high (fifteen hundred to two thousand range) with the person being very dehydrated, or even comatose. Sometimes, this is a form of presentation of diabetes and this situation must be treated quickly to save the person's life.

Diabetic Ketoacidosis frequently is not associated with a blood sugar that is very high. Sometimes, the blood sugar is no higher than the (five hundred to six hundred range) and yet the person may be in Diabetic Ketoacidosis.

WHAT IS DIABETIC KETOACIDOSIS?

Diabetic Ketoacidosis basically is a situation where the individual is unable to use sugar as fuel. Sugar is the most important fuel in the human body. If one is not able to produce insulin to break the sugar down, then one begins to use fat as fuel. The breakdown products of fat are called ketone bodies. When one uses fat as fuel, the ketone bodies accumulate in the body which can lead into a coma.

GESTATIONAL DIABETES

There is another form of Diabetes Mellitus called Gestational Diabetes. This type of diabetes is associated with pregnancy. This is a very serious condition. It has to be handled by physicians who are experts in the field of endocrinology as it relates to pregnancy. The blood sugar has to be kept much lower in women who are pregnant and diabetic because it has a direct effect on the fetus.

If this type of diabetes is not managed properly, the chances of giving birth to either a malformed or sick baby becomes very likely. It is also known that diabetic women tend to give birth to very large babies. Also, spontaneous abortion and stillbirths are both conditions that are associated with diabetes.

Gastroparesis

Other organs that are affected by diabetes are the GI tract, (the stomach), and the colon. A diabetic may develop chronic constipation because of the damage to the nerves that are associated with the proper function of the colon. Because the nerves are damaged, the proper peristalsis, or the proper movement of the colon (contraction) is impeded. Sometimes this can lead to an intestinal obstruction. In the stomach, the nerves that are associated with the lining of the stomach wall are damaged by the diabetic process. The proper contraction of the stomach musculature is therefore abnormal leading to decrease peristalsis, (food cannot go down the stomach in a normal way). The result is called Gastroparesis, which is the retention of food that cannot be digested properly, and the retention of acid leading to severe vomiting. Serious complications are associated with the inability to digest food properly. Food must be emptied out of the stomach properly into the small bowel. Obstruction can lead to devastating complications as the result of what is called Gastroparesis, which is often associated with Diabetes Mellitus.

DIABETES AND SKIN INFECTIONS

The skin can be infected very easily because diabetic individuals have a predisposition to the development of all sorts of infection and skin abscesses. A simple boil can lead to devastating infections of all kinds. So, if someone is diabetic and they have a simple skin infection, they still need to see a physician right away for appropriate antibiotics. Any infection in a diabetic is never simple. What starts out as a simple infection can lead to a catastrophe in a short time. The skin of a diabetic is to be cared for very carefully. Proper hygiene and cleansing habits have to be developed so that the individual can prevent skin infections which may later result in complications.

Type II Diabetes Mellitus is frequently associated with obesity and individuals who are obese have a great deal of difficulty with sweating resulting in a situation where they are most predisposed to the development of skin infections in the creases of the abdomen, in the groin, under the arms, etc. These individuals have to be even more careful in order to adhere to the proper hygiene, to prevent skin infections or other types of infections that can lead to abscesses that, if not treated aggressively, can lead to loss of a limb and other serious problems.

SEXUAL IMPOTENCE AND DIABETES

The underlying reason why a man becomes impotent as a result of diabetes is because of the narrowing of the vessels that carry blood to the glans penis. In order for a man to have an erection, he must have the ability to carry blood to the head of the penis. Also, he must have the ability to have properly functioning nerve impulses that are needed to stimulate the glans. The blood flow must be carried to the head of the glans penis for the erection to occur.

Because Diabetes Mellitus causes generalized arteriosclerosis and narrowing of the vessels, (that are necessary to carry blood to the glans), this results in passage (closure) and an inability of the blood to flow because of nerve damage. The result is diabetes induced impotence.

BLOOD SUGAR TEST

The most sensitive way to test for diabetes is the blood test for sugar. If the blood test for sugar is found to be elevated, then the patient is probably diabetic. However, the test for sugar in the urine is not a very accurate way to diagnose diabetes. A person's blood sugar has to be above one hundred and eighty, (the renal threshold), in order for the kidneys to allow sugar to pass. It is important to realize that the younger a person is, the more sugar passes in the urine for a given blood sugar. The older the person is, the less sugar passes. To determine if someone is diabetic, testing the urine sugar is not always very accurate. It is preferable to test for the blood sugar. If an individual has a reason to suspect that he or she might be diabetic, but the fasting blood sugar is normal, then a two hour postprandial, (a meal that contains sugar), can be performed. This is a reasonable way to diagnose if a person has hyperglycemia.

The three hour glucose tolerance test is also a test that is used to determine whether someone has glucose intolerance or not. Even more sensitive is a fasting plasma insulin level and a 2 hour plasma insulin level, and if these levels are elevated, the individual can be said to either have Diabetes Mellitus type II or will develop Diabetes Mellitus type II. In fact, this test is said to be able to determine up to a decade ahead as to whether someone is likely to become diabetic if he or she either has a parent or parents who have type II Diabetes Mellitus, according to the recent literature.

If the person presents with the classic signs of Diabetes Mellitus which are thirst, urinary frequency, and recent weight loss with general lassitude, then the diagnosis is fairly obvious. If one tests the urine there will likely be a large amount of sugar in it and acetone. The sugar in urine is graded from trace to 1+ to 4+. But, there are other conditions in medicine that can allow sugar to pass into the urine, and the person is not diabetic. This is why it is crucial to also determine the blood sugar. A diagnosis of manifested Diabetes Mellitus cannot be made unless a blood sugar test is done which is shown to be elevated and thereby consistent with the diagnosis. Two fasting blood glucose of 140 or greater MG/DL or a 2 hour post prandial blood glucose of 200 or greater are necessary for a diagnosis of Diabetes Mellitus to be made. The situation is quite different in a pregnant woman as discussed in page 9 of this chapter. In most clinical laboratories a normal blood glucose is considered to be 80 – MG/DL.

DEATH RELATED TO DIABETES

Prolongation of Symptoms

Published statistics for 1987 relating to the incidence of death resulting from Diabetes Mellitus in the United States showed that of the total 38,532 deaths, about one-sixth were African-Americans (6,497 to be exact). This is a disproportionate number. The reasons are many. The first reason is that African-Americans don't go to doctors as often as their white counterparts. And, they are not as aware of the symptoms of diabetes. By the time they go to a doctor, complications of diabetes may have occurred, often beyond repair. There could be chronic renal failure, infections that could lead to loss of a limb, or a multitude of complications, all leading to death.

Diet Management

Diet is the second reason why so many more blacks die from Diabetes Mellitus than whites. Diet is extremely important in the management of Diabetes Mellitus. Diets that are rich in carbohydrates make it very difficult to control diabetes. Carbohydrates do not cause diabetes, but they make its management more difficult. Foods that contain high carbohydrates include: sugar, syrup, rice, farina of different kinds and cereals of different kinds. These materials contain lots of carbohydrates. Fruit juices are high in sugar, and therefore, they also contain a lot of carbohydrates. All types of cakes and breads contain carbohydrates except for the low carbohydrate bread. Also, all starchy foods are high in carbohydrates. All of these food types have to be ingested in a very balanced fashion to avoid too much carbohydrate.

CONTROLLING DIABETES

Naturally, if an individual has Diabetes Mellitus, sugar must be avoided. The foods have to be measured in a fashion whereby they will be consistent with good dietary habits. Unfortunately, many Blacks who are not educated do not seem to have good diet habits. They eat what they can afford. Unfortunately, a great deal of the things that they eat are bad for them and contribute to the worsening of diseases such as Diabetes Mellitus.

Table 4.1. Different Types of Calorie Controlled Diabetic Diets

	Grams of Carbohydrates	Grams of Protein	Grams of Fat
800 calories	100	40	25
1000 calories	125	50	35
1200 calories	150	60	40
1500 calories	190	75	50
1800 calories	225	90	60
2000 calories	250	100	65
2500 calories	300	120	80
3000 calories	375	150	100

In the same vein, Blacks who are not educated as to the facts related to dietary habits, also other minorities and poor whites, don't have the means with which to go to doctors as frequently as they should. Therefore, they have symptoms that they don't understand. They don't have the money to go to clinics. Sometimes they are frustrated with the hours they have to spend in the clinic before they get seen, and they don't show up for medical evaluations. The disease is allowed to progress to a state where it becomes more advanced, much more difficult to manage, and harder for their doctor to help them. This results in the ultimate price which they must pay, death as the result of ignoring the symptoms that they were experiencing. Therefore, they allowed the process to go on too long. By the time they present themselves to a doctor, they have a serious condition such as renal failure. It is not unusual for a Black individual to go to a doctor for the first time in twenty years because of the symptoms of renal failure, only to find out the renal failure is due to diabetes.

COMPLICATIONS OF DIABETES

Diabetes Mellitus is a very peculiar disease because it is not always high blood sugar that brings the patient to the doctor. This individual can go to a doctor because he/she cannot see. They cannot see because they are diabetic. They now seek medical attention when they are already losing their eyesight and the blood sugar may only be around 140–150.

A person may go to the doctor with impotence and yet the blood sugar is only around 140–150, which is only minimally elevated. And yet, the person may already be suffering from end organ disease, (eyes, heart, kidneys), which may be affected before the blood sugar is found to be out of control. Sometimes patients have unexplained chronic abdominal pain or chronic leg pain.

Extensive evaluation may be undertaken only to find peripheral neuropathy, which is secondary to Diabetes Mellitus. But, two to three years later, the blood sugar might go out of control. Often, patients can find themselves with the effects of the diabetes before the diabetes itself is apparent, which exemplifies both the difficulties and the peculiarities of the disease.

TREATING DIABETES IN THE OFFICE SETTING

In the office setting, the juvenile diabetes subgroup is treated with Insulin. There are long-acting insulins, regular insulins, and a combination of these two. The latter is basically used to treat Juvenile Diabetes. Most of the time juvenile diabetics require insulin because the pancreatic cells that produce insulin, (the beta cells), have been destroyed. Therefore, the patients cannot produce insulin and have to receive the insulin exogenously by injection under the skin (subcutaneously) or intravenously (into the vein). Without insulin, one cannot survive because one must break down sugar to its component parts in order to live.

Sugar is needed in order to be able to carry oxygen properly to the brain, etc. Also, sugar is needed for a whole host of normal body functions. If insulin is not available to metabolize the sugar for these processes to go on, death will eventually occur.

However, Juvenile Diabetes is very difficult to treat because the blood sugars fluctuate daily, making management difficult.

Diabetes and Obesity

Obesity should be avoided at all costs, whether one has Juvenile Diabetes or Adult Onset Diabetes, because the fat cells are resistant to the effects of insulin.

When weight loss occurs, often times the amount of insulin needed for that individual decreases proportionately. Of course, the individual requires a thorough examination and explanation as to what Diabetes Mellitus is and what precautions have to be taken.

Foot Infections

The individual should not cut his/her own fingernails or toenails. One should go to a podiatrist to have that done for them. Any little nick on the foot can lead to a big infection that can lead to an ulcer which in turn can lead to the possibility of a loss of a limb.

Eye Exams

The individual also needs to have a thorough eye examination done by a physician who studied the eye as a subspecialty. This type of doctor is called an opthalmologist. The individual needs this type of doctor to examine their eyes on a regular basis. This is so because when the complications of diabetes in the eyes begin to appear, appropriate treatment can be given immediately to try to prevent the development of blindness. Please see chapter 11 under Diabetic Retinopathy.

Kidney Exams

A thorough examination of the kidney functions needs to be done by blood tests. This needs to be performed in order to have a baseline so that when these functions begin to deteriorate, appropriate comparison can be made. This allows treatment to be given quickly and adequately.

ORAL HYPOGLYCEMICS

The individual suffering from Adult Onset Diabetes has the disease because the pancreas had reached a point (because of the genetic transference of a particular gene) whereby it is failing to secrete the necessary amount of insulin needed to metabolize blood sugar. First, these individuals need to lose weight. If they are obese and lose weight, the fat cells become less resistant to the effects of the insulin, and the amount of insulin which is secreted sometimes suffices to control the blood sugar. If, in spite of losing weight, a blood sugar still remains elevated, then the doctor can provide treatment with an oral hypoglycemic agent.

The oral hypoglycemic agent stimulates the pancreas to secrete whatever insulin is left. (It is the sugar pill.) However, there is a subgroup of Adult Onset Diabetes that reaches a point where there is no longer any insulin left and the pancreas cannot be stimulated. This is what is called Type II Diabetes. The patient becomes insulin requiring at that point. This may happen at presentation, or can develop over several years of diet management. Or, after several years of a combination of diet management plus oral hypoglycemic agents, it may still develop. It is hard to determine. It is based on individual circumstances.

DIABETES TYPE II

It suffices to say that anytime from age thirty to thirty-five onward, a person can develop Diabetes Mellitus Type II. Often the patient is asked if there is a family history of diabetes. An accurate answer is sometimes difficult to ascertain. For example, a patient's mother could have died at age sixty, having never had diabetes while the patient's father, still living and at age eight-five, also has not developed the disease. Perhaps the patient's mother was carrying the gene and simply died before developing diabetes. Or, perhaps, the patient's father still has the gene but has not yet expressed it by an elevated blood sugar. It is very important that the individual understands how this process of Diabetes Mellitus Type II comes about.

When Diabetes Mellitus Type II develops an inability to respond any further to the oral hypoglycemic agents, a new modality should be considered, such as long acting insulin.

A patient should first be admitted to the hospital to get started on insulin. One never knows how an individual is going to respond to insulin treatment, or if there may be sensitivity to this medication. So, in order to avoid a disaster of hypoglycemia, introduce the concept of insulin therapy. Nurses involved in teaching diabetics how to give themselves insulin should be present. Also, the patient must learn how to self-administer the insulin. This is very important because insulin is a very dangerous medication. If one takes too much insulin, one may become hypoglycemic (low blood sugar). A low blood sugar will result in coma, seizures, and lead to death. It is crucial that a physician takes the necessary time to educate the person of the side effects of insulin and what may be expected.

Wearing Identification

On insulin, one should always carry candies and have a bracelet that identifies one as a diabetic. If the blood sugar becomes too low, it may cause confusion. Some individuals are mis-diagnosed as psychotic because of low blood sugar. Also, low blood sugar can cause a whole host of different symptoms, from psychosis to confusion—to seizures and coma. A glass of orange juice or soda will have enough sugar in it to bring one out of hypoglycemic reaction. It is very important to wear a bracelet that identifies one as a diabetic. If a police officer or some other individual finds you on the street, disabled because you have become hypoglycemic, they can look at your bracelet and see that you are diabetic and therefore will know right away that you are not someone who fell in the street due to drugs or some other thing. They can proceed to assist you in the appropriate manner and get you to the nearest emergency room so that you can be cared for appropriately to save your life.

Danger of Self-Administering Insulin

If an individual is unreliable (cannot be trusted), they may not be an appropriate candidate to receive insulin. If an individual cannot be trusted to self-administer the insulin, or doesn't have the ability to comprehend what is involved, because they may have an organic brain syndrome (that is, something is wrong with the brain and the brain is not functioning properly), they should not be allowed the opportunity to self-administer insulin because of the danger of overdose.

TREATMENT IN THE HOSPITAL SETTING

The hospital setting approach to the treatment of diabetes is more aggressive. If a person is sick enough to be admitted to the hospital on an emergency basis, and they are diabetic, they usually need insulin. The insulin will either be given subcutaneously in small doses, or it will be given intravenously as a continuous drip. Frequently, IV fluids such as normal saline or half normal saline (depending on the patients electrolytes) is administered so that the patient can be treated appropriately with insulin. The type of care given in a hospital setting for Diabetes Mellitus depends on the experience of the doctors and the competence of the hospital that is involved with the care of the patient.

Pregnant Women

For the treatment of diabetes in the pregnant woman, insulin is the treatment of choice because the blood sugar has to be kept much lower. The patient has to be kept under tight control, (called low normal glycemic control). Because any deviation in that tight control for any length of time can affect the fetus in a very negative way resulting in a malformed fetus or a fetus that is born with all sorts of other complications due to the fact that the mother did not take care of herself properly during pregnancy. This is a whole different field of obstetrics, and is best left to the obstetrician and the endocrinologists who are expert in the field to handle these particular women that are diabetic and pregnant at the same time.

Infertility

Suffice it to say, sometimes Diabetes Mellitus itself can lead to infertility resulting in difficulties in getting pregnant. This is something to keep in mind if a woman is having difficulty getting pregnant. One of the things that has to be looked at is the concept as to whether or not she may or may not be diabetic.

SENSITIVITY TO INSULIN

Diabetes Mellitus is a very serious disease. It is divided into two types: Juvenile Diabetes, known as Type I Diabetes and Adult Onset Diabetes, known as Type II Diabetes. An individual who has chronic pancreatitis as a result of alcohol abuse, let's say, can have Type II like Diabetes Mellitus. Or, an individual who may be sent to the hospital with non-ketotic hyperosmolar state with a very high blood sugar and coma. These individuals are extremely sensitive to insulin. It is important that fluid be administered aggressively and insulin is administered very carefully, because it can lower the blood sugar precipitously. This must be avoided. Once fluid has been administered, the insulin should be given slowly and carefully to lower the blood sugar.

These individuals frequently and typically turn out to require no insulin at all once their condition is corrected and can be managed with sometimes just on diet alone, or sometimes with very small doses of insulin. Of course, sometimes they go on to require regular treatment with insulin etc. There are many different varieties that can be seen.

DIET AND INSULIN

As far as diet is concerned, it is the key. Diet is always very important when someone is diabetic. A low carbohydrate diet is crucial. In some individuals a 1000 calorie diet may be appropriate. In another, 1200 calories may be appropriate. In still another, it may be 1500 calories. In another subgroup, 1800 calories, especially in men, can be appropriate. So, the important thing to understand is that the ingestion of carbohydrates can complicate the condition named Diabetes Mellitus and obesity makes this condition extremely difficult to deal with because these individuals who are diabetic and also obese have a resistance to insulin, either insulin administered exogenously or insulin that is being secreted endogenously by the body itself.

What is interesting is that the insulin is an anabolic agent, meaning that it is an agent that makes you gain weight by itself. So if a person is obese, the more insulin you give them, the more obese they are likely to become, raising the need for insulin even more. Insulin tends to increase a person's appetite even more. So, it is important to understand that the idea is not to just keep giving insulin to these people, but rather to try to get them to lose weight so that the need for insulin will be less and less, rather than more and more.

DIABETES AND EDUCATION, KEY TO MANAGEMENT

Diabetes Mellitus is a multisystem disease. Precautions have to be taken so the eyes can be safeguarded, the kidneys, the heart, the legs, the skin and a whole host of other things need to be done. By getting in contact with the American Diabetic Association to get literature, the individual can become very familiar, very educated in the management of diabetes and how it should be treated and handled.

Controlling Diet

It is crucial to take the time to choose the proper foods to eat, regardless of one's economic situation. Time should be taken for careful selection of food that will enhance one's health rather than harm it.

Controlling Blood Sugar

It is known fact that the better the blood sugar is controlled in a diabetic person, the less the complications of the diabetes, anywhere from the eye complications, to the kidney complications, etc. The idea is to try to control the blood sugar so that the end organ damage will be limited.

LIVING WITH DIABETES

In summary, once diabetic, always diabetic. But, once diabetic does not mean necessarily always treatment for diabetes. If the diet is good, then a so-called sugar pill or oral hypoglycemic may not be needed. If the diet is well-controlled one may not need insulin. But, if insulin is needed, one should not be afraid nor be ashamed to take it because it is needed to stay alive. The important thing is education and the understanding that a disease that is not curable is treatable. It is a lifetime disease that one has to learn how to live with. Learn how to get emotionally involved in the disease to help manage its conditions. Become a self-expert on how to manage this disease. One can lead a perfectly normal life with Diabetes Mellitus if one understands the disease, the complications, and, how to properly react to these complications in an informed and correct manner.

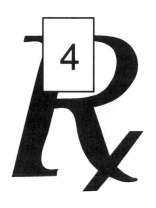

HEART DISEASE AND ITS ASSOCIATED PROBLEMS IN AFRICAN-AMERICANS

CHAPTER OUTLINE

HEART DISEASE INCREASING AMONG BLACKS

In the United States, heart disease is the Number One cause of death in all segments of the population. However, the incidence of heart disease associated with coronary artery disease has been decreasing, in the white population, for unknown reasons. It is believed that the change in lifestyle, diet, exercise, etc. may be playing a role in this decrease.

On the other hand, heart disease in the African-American population is increasing at an alarming rate. Heart disease resulting in heart attack, stroke, or both is now the number one cause leading to death in African-Americans. The reasons for this are probably due to the more stressful situations of life, poor living conditions, and the fact that African-Americans are not getting adequate medical attention.

WHAT IS HEART DISEASE?

Heart disease is a general term which applies to a number of heart dysfunctions. The two most common forms are: 1) arteriosclerotic heart disease (which leads to occlusion of the coronary arteries causing angina—leading to chest pain—leading to heart attack); and 2) coronary artery disease (which may lead to ischemia of the myocardium—causing chronic ischemic heart disease resulting in chronic chest pain, ischemic cardiomyopathy, all which may lead to congestive heart failure).

ARTERIOSCLEROTIC HEART DISEASE

The most common form of heart disease is arteriosclerotic heart disease. This disease is associated with the development of plaques in the arteries around the heart which causes the narrowing of these arteries. This impedes the passage of blood, and thereby impedes the delivery of oxygen to the mus-

cles of the heart. Blood carries oxygen and has to be able to pass through the vessels, so the muscles of the heart can function properly. However, there are different degrees of narrowing of the vessels, from 10% narrowing to 100% narrowing.

SYMPTOMS AND RISK FACTORS OF HEART DISEASE

Sometimes, a significant narrowing of these vessels is present, and yet the patient may or may not be symptomatic. For example, he/she could have a massive heart attack, and yet there may be no symptoms, or there may be symptoms which are ignored or thought to be insignificant. So, if one has a family member, i.e. father, mother with coronary disease and/or heart attack, this positive family history could be a risk factor. Also, a high cholesterol level, obesity, and smoking cigarettes are all major risk factors. So, if one is the age of 35 onward and experiences a shortness of breath or a tightness in the chest when walking, there may be a problem. If pain develops down the left shoulder, and the arm becomes numb, this may also be symptomatic. Again, the physician will try to determine by the clinical history what is significant.

DETERMINING HEART ASSOCIATED CHEST PAIN

There are a multitude of facts needed to determine whether the patient does have a condition of heart associated chest pain.

Sometimes, it may only be indigestion that may manifest symptoms of a serious heart condition. There is a form of heart attack, (an inferior wall myocardial infarction), which is almost always associated with nausea and vomiting. Nausea and vomiting therefore may be symptoms of an acute heart attack without one realizing it. So, if there are chest pains associated with nausea and vomiting, a cold sweat, and a feeling of dizziness, these symptoms could be evidence of an acute heart attack.

Of course, nausea and vomiting could mean a whole host of other things, such as gallbladder disease, peptic ulcer disease of the stomach, or acute gastroenteritis. But, leave the diagnosis to your doctor, or go to an emergency room and try to be evaluated (i.e. an electrocardiogram). But, one should be aware that a negative electrocardiogram does not always mean that one hasn't experienced a heart attack. It is the total, family and personal history and the physical exam that decides whether or not there should be suspicion for a heart attack, or that one is about to occur. Or, a determination may be established that it is an ulcer disease or a gastroenteritis. An experienced physician will make the decision accurately and promptly.

CORONARY ARTERY DISEASE

Plaque

Occlusion of the coronary artery occurs because of plaque. In its native form, these vessels have a lumen that is very clean and smooth. If, for instance, the person is hypertensive, (high blood pressure), the sheer increased pressure of the blood passing through the vessel can cause the vessel to lose its integrity—leading to the deposition of plaques.

Clots

If one has high cholesterol, cholesterol plaques begin to form within the lumen of the vessels, trapping platelets and other material, as they pass through. These plaques start

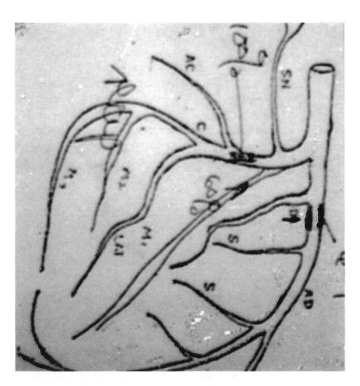

Figure 4.1. Plaques in left coronary artery. (small arrows showing plaques in left coronary artery 60% occlusion in a 49 year-old male with high cholesterol)

37

to form clots. Sometimes, the vessel not only narrows, which prevents blood from passing through (which leads to ischemia), but also there can be an actual rupture of one of these plaques. This can lead to bleeding within the vessel, which may cause a formation of clots which may also cause an acute heart attack.

RISK FACTORS OF CORONARY ARTERY DISEASE

Therefore, to prevent a heart attack, the risk factors are very important to take into consideration. The problem with Blacks is that they are not paying attention to the risk factors. Smoking is on the rise. Alcohol abuse is on the rise. Also, any increase in alcohol drinking may increase the incidence of myocardial disease. Also, alcoholism may cause an increase in coronary artery disease because of an increase of high blood pressure. Drinking may cause a state of agitation, and any persistent state of agitation may cause blood pressure to increase, which also can lead to coronary artery disease.

Poor Diet

One of the most important issues is diet. One that is rich in saturated fat, is also a predisposing factor to coronary artery disease. Certainly, pork, beef, and other high cholesterol content foods (the vast majority of Blacks eat because of habit or poverty) predispose them to high cholesterol. This, in turn, leads to coronary artery disease.

Most Blacks in the inner cities don't have the full opportunity to go to the big supermarkets to shop for choice foods. They have to buy from the local little stores where they can. Usually when they buy there, it is one and a half to two times more expensive than they would buy in a bigger supermarket in the suburb, but it is still not very good food. It is full of carbohydrates, full of cholesterol, and most of the time full of salt causing problems for the heart.

Hyperlipidemia

(High Cholesterol, High Triglyceride, Low HDL, High LDL)

Genetic Predisposition

(i.e., If mother or father has coronary artery disease, chances of one developing coronary artery disease is high)

Obesity

In addition, the lack of exercise (because Blacks in the U.S. are in no condition to have the facilities to get involved in an exercise program) makes obesity a major problem in Black women, and for that matter also in Black men, resulting in another form of risk factor for coronary artery disease and heart attacks.

Hypertension

The other major risk factor of course is hypertension. Essential hypertension is very high in the Black community. Most of it goes untreated, and a significant segment of it, when it is being treated, is being treated improperly. Many physicians do not know how to treat hypertension appropriately in Blacks. Some are treated with inappropriate medications and are not given diuretics. In addition, some are given a whole host of medications that have no relationship to helping the blood pressure go down, (such as, the beta blockers, the ACE inhibitors, and the calcium channel blockers). These medications may be good as antihypertensive medication—but not as a single medication by themselves in Blacks.

Even if these medications bring the blood pressure down in a black person, as a single medication this decrease would only be transient. The blood pressure will eventually readjust itself and rise to an abnormal level again.

Therefore, the most important thing is that when the blood pressure is not treated properly, it remains elevated and the result is an increase in coronary artery disease which in turn can lead to myocardial ischemic disease leading to heart attack and death.

Smoking

The nicotine and possibly other chemical substances in tobacco cause the development of atherosclarotic disease in vessels around the heart resulting in coronary artery disease.

EVALUATION OF CHEST PAIN—ACUTE MYOCARDIAL INFARCTION SETTING

What To Do if Experiencing Chest Pain

The first thing one should do, of course, is to go to a physician. Let him/her examine you, take a thorough assessment of the implications. If the pain is increasing and decreasing and the doctor does not recommend hospitalization immediately, then an evaluation needs to be undertaken. This includes an evaluation of the blood to check blood chemistries to see if there are any predisposing factors such as high cholesterol, or anemia. Once this is done, a chest x-ray is necessary (discomfort in the chest could mean another disease such as cancer of the lung). Cancer of the lung can manifest itself with chest pain. Also, fluid around the lung can present itself as discomfort in the chest such as pleuritis, (inflammation of the lining of the lung, the pleura). This is why it is important to have a chest x-ray.

If one has a cardiomyopathy (an enlarged heart) secondary to some underlying disease of the myocardium, a viral infection (that you may or may not know about), can lead to chest pain.

EMERGENCY ROOM PROCEDURE—IDEAL SETTING

If one has chest pain and is taken to the emergency room, he/she should be evaluated by a physician. The questions to be asked are—

1. How long have you been having the pain?
2. The location of the chest pain
3. The quality of the pain
4. The severity of the pain
5. The types of pain, Is the pain dull? Is the pain sharp, knifelike? Is the pain like a pressure in the chest, like someone sitting on your chest?
6. Does the pain radiate to the left arm or left shoulder?
   Does it hurt when you move your left shoulder?
7. Does it hurt when I press on your chest with my fingers?
8. Does it hurt when you take a deep breath? (pleuritic)
9. Is the pain associated with shortness of breath and/or sweating? (diaphoresis)

(Pleuritic chest pain implies pain coming from the lungs such as pneumonia, pleuritis or pulmonary embolism).

All these are very important things to know because a decision has to be made to determine if there has been a heart attack, and how many hours ago it may have happened, or is the patient having unstable angina but a heart attack has not yet occurred (pre-infarction angina).

At This Point

1. An EKG is needed
2. Portable chest x-ray
3. Nasal oxygen ought to be given, 3 liters per minute

4. A trial of sub-lingual nitroglycerine if the blood pressure is either normal or elevated. If the patient responds to the sub-lingual nitroglycerine in a few minutes, this usually means that the patient's chest pain is probably due to coronary insufficiency.

An evaluation of the EKG may point in a direction that an acute myocardial infarction has occurred by showing abnormalities in T waves, ST T waves and Q waves changes. It is important to remember that a patient who is about to have a heart attack may present with a perfectly normal EKG. If it is determined based on clinical findings and judgment that this patient is suffering from pre-infarction angina, the modern treatment then, is an infusion of heparin via IV drip and aspirin by mouth in conjunction with nitrates either by mouth, by paste on the chest wall or by IV depending on the severity of the pain. In this setting it is wise to also use a Beta-Blocker. It is important to make sure that there are no contraindications to—

1. Aspirin
2. Heparin
3. Beta-Blocker

If the EKG shows evidence that an acute myocardial infarction has occurred and it is determined that it probably occurred less than four hours before presentation then a t-PA (tissue plasminogen activator) ought to be given to dissolve the clot within the coronary artery thereby limiting the size of the myocardial infarction. According to the literature, this procedure leads to significant increase in survival from acute myocardial infarction. t-PA is most effective when infused 1–3 hours after an acute myocardial infarction has occurred.

t-PA is made by recombinant DNA technology and needs fibrin as a mediator for activation of plasminogen, which selectively mediates thrombolysis at the site of clot for-mation with only slight systemic fibrinolysis. (Only very little amounts of t-PA enter the blood circulation, which is why it is a very safe medication, though a very expensive one).

Streptokinase can also be used to dissolve clots in the setting of an acute myocardial infarction, but it has more side effects and there are more contraindications to using it.

DETERMINING A HEART ATTACK

Elevation of Enzymes

When the muscle of the heart is damaged, it secretes certain enzymes into the blood. The CPK (creatinine phosphokinase) is the first enzyme that becomes elevated. The second enzyme is SGOT (serum glutamic oxaloacetic transaminase), and the third is the LDH (Lactic dehydrogenase) which are secreted in sequence. These bloods should be drawn for three separate days to see if they are elevated. If they are elevated and the elevation of the CPK is associated with a fraction of the CPK that comes from the muscle of the heart, (the MB fraction), then the patient has had a heart attack. If, however, the elevation of the CPK is due to skeletal muscle, then there will be a 100% MM. This means that the muscle comes from the skeletal muscle and a heart attack has not occurred. A heart attack has occurred if the muscle of the myocardium has been damaged, and then there is an elevation of the MB fraction of the total CPK. At this point, the percentage determining the height of the CPK is a good determinant of how massive the heart attack has been. This is very important because at this point, it should be determined that the EKG is abnormal. This is associated with certain findings on an EKG that are associated with muscle damage of the heart. If the patient has an elevation in their CPK, the MB fraction is elevated, the SGOT is elevated, and the LDH is elevated, one can diagnose a heart attack. Hopefully, it is an uncomplicated heart attack with no cardiac arrhythmias. If the rhythm of the heart remains normal, breathing remains normal, and there is no accumulating fluid in the lungs, then there is no congestive heart failure, no persistent chest pain, then this is called an un-completed heart attack.

However, the worst case scenario is a heart attack that has actually ruptured the muscle of the heart. This results almost always in death.

Other things that may happen to the heart such as a rupture of the vessel of the chordae tendineae which is another one of the highly sophisticated things that can happen to the heart which can lead to congestive heart failure.

NEED FOR LIDOCAINE

If one has a heart attack at home, an ambulance should be called, and it should be equipped with Lidocaine. People who receive Lidocaine on the way to the hospital (prophylactically) survive more often than those who receive it after they reach the hospital. Lidocaine treats cardiac arrhythmias such as VPC's. These can lead to ventricular tachycardia, which, if sustained, is life threatening. The heart will just simply stop functioning and death will occur. Lidocaine is also used for other types of arrhythmias.

VENTRICULAR FIBRILLATION

When a patient has had a heart attack, the patient dies because of the abnormality of the rhythm of the heart. The muscle is damaged so much that it leads to abnormalities such as acute congestive heart failure (pulmonary edema). During a heart attack, the patient can also develop ventricular fibrillation. This is when the heart loses its contractibility which is also life threatening.

It is very important that one understands that a heart attack has occurred and it is the complications that lead to death. Therefore, the sooner one gets to a hospital, the sooner appropriate treatment can be administered.

HEART BLOCK

Sometimes the electrical system of the heart fails causing a bundle branch block or heart block, known as 1st degree, 2nd degree, 3rd degree heart block. These types of heart blocks are sometimes so severe that an emergency pacemaker has to be inserted in the patient's heart in order to sustain the electrical system of the heart. Of course, there is a disease of the elderly called sick sinus syndrome; whereby, because of the aging of the electrical system of the heart, heart block can develop causing dizziness and the patient has to be treated by a pacemaker inserted inside the heart to take over the electrical function of the heart.

HEART ATTACK AND THE DIABETIC

It is important to mention here that for individuals who are diabetic, they have to be extra careful. Not only does the diabetes predispose them to coronary artery disease which can lead to a heart attack, but also these individuals who are diabetic have a propensity to have painless heart attacks, (having a heart attack but no pain associated with it). Therefore, they have to be more the vigilant in trying to get to the doctor as quickly as possible. This is very important because if a major cardiac problem occurs, and they don't realize it, they die without even realizing they were having a heart attack. This happens because diabetics have damaged nerve fibers. Since these nerve fibers are damaged, they often times do not respond to pain as readily as non-diabetics do. So, it is very important that someone who is diabetic, and in the age group that is prone to having heart attacks, be ever careful and try to determine when one may be occurring. Something as simple as having a very bad stomach upset and/or feeling dizzy, may be the first indication that the patient needs to be taken to the hospital right away. If a diabetic is not feeling well, it could be associated also with either high or low blood sugar.

THE NEED FOR ANTICOAGULATION AND HEART DISEASES

If a heart attack occurs, in the acute setting the individual may benefit from treatment with heparin. In particular, if the individual develops congestive heart failure which is associated with a heart attack; then heparin may prevent the development of pulmonary embolism, or phlebitis. Because of the fact that the individual is forced to remain at bed rest which predisposes them to the development of a hypercoaguable state. As mentioned before in this chapter, heparin is not only indicated in the preinfarction state, but also heparin has been documented to be helpful in preventing the development of intramural clots in the setting of an acute myocardial infarction. In valvular heart disease such as mitral stenosis with associated atrial fibrillation; Coumadin is used by mouth to thin the blood, preventing clots from forming on the abnormal valves. If not treated in this fashion it can lead to strokes. Most recently, the literature recommends that non-valvular associated atrial fibrillation should also be treated with coumadin to prevent strokes.

STRESS TESTING AFTER HEART ATTACK PRIOR TO GOING HOME

After several days in the hospital, assuming that there are no complications, often times the patient is encouraged to get up as quickly as possible. Before the patient goes home, it is a good idea for the patient to have the so-called low level stress test. This should give the physician an idea as to what level of activity the patient will or will not be able to do at home. This enables the physician to tell the patient what he/she can and can not do based on the result of this test. It tells what actual level of stress the heart is now capable of handling.

GATED BLOOD POOL SCAN AFTER A HEART ATTACK

When the patient is about to go home, a rest gated blood pool (MUGA) scan should be done and an ejection fraction obtained. This helps to determine how well the muscle is functioning. To a degree, this test can be used to plan the immediate future for the patient.

CHEST PAIN SYNDROME

When a patient presents to the doctor with chest pain, there are a long list of different conditions the doctor must think about in order to determine the cause of the chest pain.

1. *Heart Disease*
   a) Acute myocardial infarction
   b) Angina pectoris
   c) Viral pericarditis
   d) Mitral value prolapse
2. *Pulmonary Disease*
   a) Acute pulmonary embolism
   b) Pneumonia
   c) Lung cancer
   d) Pleuritis
3. *Acute Costochondritis*
4. *Acute Gall Bladder Disease*
5. *Acute Peptic Ulcer Disease*

PULMONARY DISEASE AS A CAUSE OF CHEST PAIN

The most acute conditions to think of that can cause acute chest pain as a result of pulmonary problem are:—

a) Acute pulmonary embolism
b) Pneumonia
c) Viral infection resulting in pleuritis
d) In patients with sickle cell disease, acute painful crisis vs acute chest pain syndrome
e) Lung cancer

ACUTE COSTOCHONDRITIS

A chest pain syndrome can simply be due to costochondritis, (an inflammation of the ribs and the muscles within the ribs). This can be very painful and very distressing. Costochondritis is reasonably common, but many people have wound up in a coronary care unit believing that they were having a heart attack when in fact it was costochondritis.

These types of conditions (costochondritis and pericarditis) respond to aspirin (an anti-inflammatory medication). They also respond to medications such as Indocin which is also an anti-inflammatory type mediation. But, again, one needs a doctor with good judgement. Certainly one wouldn't prescribe aspirin for someone whose chest pain is due to an ulcer. This could lead to a catastrophe resulting in bleeding. Also, one wouldn't prescribe Indocin for someone who has an ulcer causing a chest pain; again this would be dangerous.

As to when and how one decided to do these things, that's when experience comes into the picture. Medical practice is a combination of knowledge and experience. It is really an art form. Experience is its essence. One just can't pick up a book, read it, and them practice medicine. One really has to have years of training and practice so that one can determine the nuances of when and when not to respond. This is where the master clinician is essential.

ACUTE GALL BLADDER DISEASE

Acute gall bladder disease can sometime presents with chest pain that simulates an acute cardiac event. Sometimes even with EKG changes, that can mislead one into believing that one is dealing with coronary insufficiency.

At times, the individual may even respond to sub-lingual nitro glycerine. Therefore, if no other cause can be found to explain the chest discomfort, an abdominal sonogram should be done to rule out the possibility of gall bladder disease.

ACUTE PEPTIC ULCER DISEASE

Reasonably, frequently, acute chest discomfort can be the result of acute peptic ulcer disease. If no other explanation can be found to explain the chest discomfort then, a trial of H2 blocker ought to be started and then an upper GI series done to rule out the possibility of peptic ulcer disease being the cause of the chest pain.

EVALUATION OF CHEST PAIN IN A SETTING WHERE A HEART ATTACK HAS NOT OCCURRED

When it has been determined that a heart attack has not occurred in a patient who presented to the hospital with chest pain, and yet the possibility is that the patient may have underlying heart disease, and or other condition as a cause of the chest pain still exist then several tests must be done in order to determine the reason for the chest pain.

THE DIFFERENT TESTS TO DO IN EVALUATING NON-HEART ATTACK TYPE CHEST PAIN

1. Echocardiogram
2. Cardiac Stress Tests
   a) Stress gated blood pool (known also as stress MUGA)
   b) Treadmill stress test
   c) Thalium stress test
   d) Persantine thalium stress test

DESCRIPTION OF ECHOCARDIOGRAM

The echocardiogram is done by placing a probe on the chest wall around the heart which is attached to an echocardiogram machine. The echocardiogram enables the physician to see inside the heart thereby being able to evaluate the valvular abnormalities and/or muscular abnormalities involving the different chambers of the heart. The sac around the heart called the pericardium can be thoroughly evaluated looking for fluid and other abnormalities in it. Doppler-echocardiogram maximizes the sensitivity of the echocardiogram. If cardial muscular damage has occurred, the echocardiogram is capable of determining that.

OTHER CARDIAC CONDITIONS IN WHICH ECHOCARDIOGRAM IS USED AS A VALUABLE DIAGNOSTIC TOOL

1. Mitral Valve Prolapse
2. Pericarditis
3. Pericardial Effusion
4. Valvular Heart Disease
5. Cardiomyopathy
6. Bacterial Endocarditis

STRESS GATED BLOOD POOL (MUGA)

Stress gated blood pool (known also as stress MUGA) evaluates the heart in a different manner. Not only utilizing exercise, but by also using a small amount of nuclear substance injected simultaneously into the blood. Certain essential numbers can be determined such as the ejection fraction of the heart. This allows the physician to have a sum total of the function of the heart. An ejection fraction that is 40% or less indicates that something is wrong with the heart, but, an ejection fraction that is 60% or greater is considered normal.

An ejection fraction is something that relates the sum total of the work that the heart is able to perform at a given time. It evaluates the muscles of the heart. It is not specific, but it gives a good description of the performance of the heart.

During this test, the muscle of the heart can actually be seen, and if there is a defect in the muscle of the heart, this also can be seen.

TREADMILL STRESS TEST

Before a cardiac catheterization is recommended, in the process of evaluating the chest pain, ordinarily one would first do the treadmill stress test. If the treadmill stress test is normal, but the doctor does not have a complete diagnosis on why the chest pain continues and a trial of medication for angina has not helped, then it is a good idea to examine the gallbladder. An abdominal sonogram would be performed to rule out gallstones. This is a very simple procedure where a probe is placed on the abdomen. The sonogram is performed, after fasting from foods & liquids, usually the next morning. At the same sitting, if necessary, if the abdominal sonogram is negative, then one can have an upper GI series performed. At this time, the stomach can be evaluated to see if there is a stomach ulcer, or possibly, a hiatal hernia (associated refluxing toward the upper stomach and throat leading to a bitter taste). These things can all cause chest discomfort. It is not at all unusual for one to have severe chest pain and be admitted to the hospital coronary care unit, only to find out it was due to an ulcer.

THALIUM STRESS TEST

There are two types of Thalium stress tests. One type is done with an exercise component and the other type is done at rest. Thalium is a nuclear tracer which is similar to potassium in its chemical properties. The basis of the Thalium Stress Tests is the following— Heart muscles that have died and become scarred after a myocardial infarction (heart attack) are not able to pick up potassium from the blood circulation. However, viable heart muscle is capable of taking up potassium from the circulation. Therefore, if Thalium is injected into the blood of an individual the Thalium is expected to be picked up by viable heart muscles. On the other hand, if the muscles have died and become scarred as a result of a heart attack, they will not pick up the Thalium. Using these facts as a basis, Thalium is injected into the blood stream during a cardiac stress test and pictures of the heart is displayed during the exercise and also at rest. If a defect is noted in the muscle of the heart during the stress of exercise and that defect remains persistent during the rest period of the test, then that means that the defective area was not able to pick up the Thalium because that is an area of dead heart muscle, thus documenting that a previous myocardial infarction has occurred (this person has had a heart attack in the past). On the other hand, if the abnormality noted in the heart muscle during exercise, and that abnormality disappeared during the rest period of the Thalium Stress Test, then that means the individual is having coronary insufficiency manifesting as angina pectoris (manifesting as chest pain clinically). The reason why the abnormality appears during the exercise is because of narrowing of coronary arteries due to plaques impeding the delivery of oxygen to that area when the demand for oxygen is at its maximum because of the stress of exercise and yet it cannot be delivered in sufficient amount. At rest the oxygen demand decreases and the area now becomes normalized with a defect that was seen having disappeared. Single photon emission computed tomography test (SPECT) is used to increase the accuracy of the test.

PERSANTINE THALIUM STRESS TEST

The second type of Thalium Stress Test is called the Persantine Thalium Stress Test. This test is devised to accommodate individuals who, for any number of reasons, show contra indication for exercise cardiac stress testing (the indications may be due to excessive obesity, chronic bronchitis, herniated lumbar disc, severe arthritis of the knees and legs and a variety of other serious medical problems such as recurrent chest pains). Persantine is used along with Thalium to stress the heart itself but no other part of the human anatomy, and the information obtained is similarly interpreted as that of the first Thalium described above and the results have the same clinical implications. This is based on the fact that dipyridamole (Persantine) is used either by mouth or intravenously to cause vaso dilatation of the coronary arteries; then the Thalium is injected allowing identification of abnormalities in the muscle of the heart using single photon emission computed tomography (SPECT) imaging.

CORONARY ANGIOGRAM

If any one of these tests show an abnormality suggestive of coronary artery disease and the doctor is concerned about it, then the coronary angiogram ought to be considered if the clinical setting is appropriate.

The coronary angiogram is done by injecting a dye in the groin using the femoral artery and a catheter is connected to the chambers of the heart. This process can display the vessels around the heart enabling the doctor to see if there are occlusions in them. This is really the best method for determining if something is wrong with the coronary arteries. But, this is an invasive procedure, and it is not performed unless there is good reason to suspect coronary disease. However, other problems with the valves of the heart may also warrant for this procedure. This procedure has a small percentage of risk associated with it, but it is a crucial test when needed. It is just about impossible to get the needed information any other way.

If the stress test is abnormal, the coronary angiogram is abnormal. It shows different degrees of occlusion in either one vessel, two vessels, or three vessels.

SURGICAL TREATMENT OPTIONS

Angioplasty or Coronary Bypass

The next step will depend on whether or not the ventricle is functioning well, pumping well, and the ejection fraction is good. The doctor should try to offer treatment that will be ultimately needed to resolve the problem. One may become a candidate for an angioplasty. This is basically cardiac catheterization which removes some of the plaques from the vessels. The first step of this procedure re-opens the vessels without having to perform major open heart surgery.

Next, the cardiologist and the cardiac surgeons may recommend coronary bypass to resolve the problem. However, there is no definitive evidence that coronary bypass surgery prolongs life in the aggregate, though individual patients' life may be prolonged by it. There is definitive evidence that coronary bypass relieves symptoms such as angina, and shortness of breath, thereby improving the overall quality of life in patients who have undergone the surgical procedure.

MEDICAL TREATMENT PLAN

If cardiac catheterization is either refused because the myocardium is so bad and the ejection fraction is too low, i.e. less than 30%, or the patient refuses to accept surgery, then medications must be prescribed to relieve the symptoms of angina and/or congestive heart failure. There are different ways of treating these conditions. The doctor and the patient have to sit down and formulate a treatment plan that will accurately determine the need of the patient.

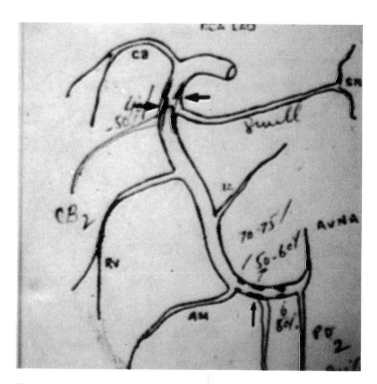

Figure 4.2. Big arrows showing 40 to 50 percent of the proximal portion of the right coronary artery. Small arrow showing 70–75 percent occlusion of the distal right coronary artery. This right coronary artery has diffuse atherosclerotic changes in other areas.

OTHER CARDIAC CONDITIONS THAT CAUSE CHEST PAIN

VIRAL PERICARDITIS

Viral pericarditis is an inflammation of the sac (within which the heart is contained) which is the pericardium leading to pericarditis. Pericarditis sometimes is self-limiting; but other times, it can be chronic leading to a serious condition that can result in death. Most often, however, it is resolved over several months with appropriate treatment. Pericarditis causes severe chest pain.

TREATMENTS OF PERICARDITIS

The treatments of pericarditis are—

a)   bed rest
b)   aspirin or Indocin

VIRAL MYOCARDITIS

The heart can be infected by a variety of organisms such as virus, bacteria, fungi, different parasites leading to disease of the heart. Viral myocarditis is very common. This is an inflam-

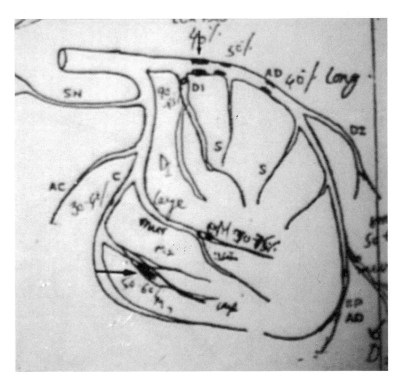

Figure 4.3. Small arrow shows 40% occlusion of the proximal left anterior descending artery. There is a 30% occlusion of the LAD in its proximal portion just before the first major septal artery and also there is a 40% occlusion in the midst portion of the LAD.

Big arrow shows 50 to 60 percent occlusion of the epical diagonal branch of the left coronary artery. There are several areas of diffuse atherosclerotic changes involving this left coronary artery.

These occlusive changes of these coronary arteries were seen in a 42 year old man with hypertension and high cholesterol who also smokes cigarettes.

mation of the muscle of the heart as a result of infection due to a virus, and/or fungus.

TREATMENTS OF MYOCARDITIS

The treatments of myocarditis are—

a) bed rest
b) aspirin or Indocin

MITRAL VALVE PROLAPSE

There is a condition called mitral valve prolapse which is very common in North America. It used to be believed that mitral valve prolapse was associated with people who were very tall, such as people with Marfan's syndrome. In fact, it is not at all necessary to be tall in order to have mitral valve prolapse. In fact, since there are more short people than tall people in the population, one has to assume that the mitral valve prolapse is seen in more short individuals than tall individuals.

Mitral valve prolapse may be a very serious condition. In some cases it is very mild; but at other times, it is very serious where the mitral valve is prolapsing onto itself—resulting in shortness of breath, chest pain, and sometimes very lethal arrhythmias, all can lead to collapse and death.

TREATMENTS OF MITRAL VALVE PROLAPSE

Medical treatments of mitral valve prolapse are—

a) beta blockers such as Inderal
b) non-steroidal anti-inflammatory drugs such as Motrin
c) in rare instances surgical treatment may be necessary

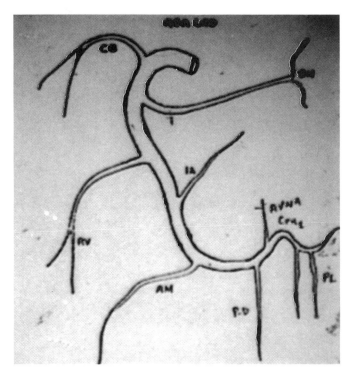

Figure 4.4. A normal right coronary artery.

SUBACUTE BACTERIAL ENDOCARDITIS OR ACUTE BACTERIAL ENDOCARDITIS

Another serious form of heart disease that is afflicting Blacks in the inner city is the infection of the heart associated with drug addiction called acute bacterial endocarditis, or subacute bacterial endocarditis. When an individual is using IV drugs and in the process of injecting the drug into the vein, organisms, bacteria, or fungus get injected into the blood stream, and get deposited on the valves of the heart, the mitral valve, aortic valve, the tricuspid valve, eating away at the valves causing bacterial endocarditis. This can lead to decomposition of the heart function, eventually causing death. This is the direct result of IV drug addiction.

MEDICAL TREATMENT OF SUBACUTE AND ACUTE ENDOCARDITIS

If one suspects subacute bacterial endocarditis, then one has to draw blood cultures and start empiric IV antibiotics pending the result of the blood cultures. Definitive antibiotic treatment will be determined based on the result of the blood cultures. An echocardiogram is very important in that it evaluated the valves of the heart and also evaluate whether or not there is vegetation on the valves of the heart.

However, most of all is the frequent examination of the heart and the lungs to ascertain whether or not the patient is decompensating or not from a cardiovascular stand point; which usually means the appearance of

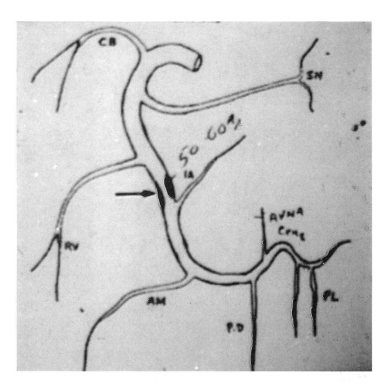

Figure 4.5. Big arrow shows 50 to 60 percent occlusion in the mid portion of a right coronary artery.

a heart murmur and signs of congestive heart failure. When these occur, then the cardiac surgeon team must be called immediately to evaluate the patient for the possibility of valve replacement in order to save the patient's life.

HIV TYPE I VIRUS AND HEART DISEASE

The heart can also become infected by the HIV Type I virus, so-called AIDS virus, also causing pericarditis, myocarditis, leading to dysfunction of the heart that can also lead to the demise of the individual.

HEMOCHROMATOSIS, IRON AND CARDIOMYOPATHY

There are two types of Hemochromatosis.

a) Idiopathic Hemochromatosis

b) Secondary Hemochromatosis

Primary hemochromatosis is a genetically transmitted metabolic condition in which the intestinal epithelial cell loses the ability to regulate absorption of iron. Individuals with this condition over absorb iron (up to 15 times more than normal) causing too much iron to enter into the body. The estimated incidence of Idiopathic Hemochromatosis in the U.S. population is said to be 0.005%. Therefore, about 10% of the U.S. population are carriers of this abnormal gene.

Secondary Hemochromatosis is due to dyserythropoeisis (i.e. abnormal hemoglobin causing red blood cells to die too soon releasing iron into the blood). Examples of conditions that cause Secondary Hemochromatosis are:

1. Beta Thalassemia

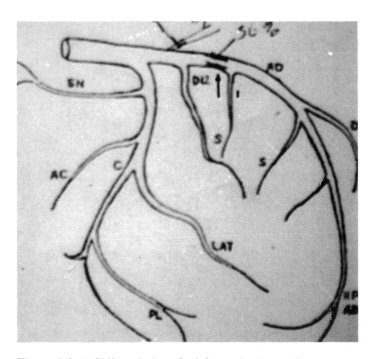

Figure 4.6. A 50% occlusion of a left anterior descending coronary artery both in a patient with high cholesterol and hypertension.

2. Alpha Thalassemia
3. Sickle Cell Disease
4. Hereditary Spherocytosis
5. Other Chronic Hemolytic Diseases

OTHER WAYS TO DIAGNOSE IDIOPATHIC HEMOCHROMATOSIS IS

1. Do serum ferritin and if the serum ferritin is 500 NG/ML or greater, that by definition is Idiopathic Hemochromatosis if no other explanations can be found to explain the high serum ferritin, such as infection, inflammation or abnormal hemoglobins.
2. Do a Magnetic Resonance Imaging (MRI) of the liver looking for iron deposition. If the MRI is positive for iron deposition in the liver, this calls for institutional treatment to remove the excess iron in the body to prevent diseases such as:

a. Cardiomyopathy (enlargement of the heart) secondary to deposition of iron in the heart muscles.
b. Diabetes Mellitus secondary to deposition of iron in the pancreas.
c. Cirrhosis of the liver secondary to deposition of iron in the liver.
d. To prevent the possibility of primary cancer of the liver (hepatocellular carcinoma of the liver) as a result of the toxic nature of iron.
See the chapter on anemia for further discussion on Hemochromatosis.

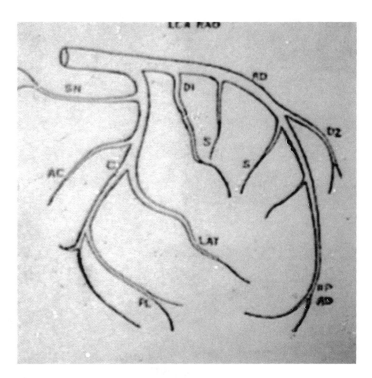

Figure 4.7. A normal left coronary artery.

Cardiomyopathy which resulted from Hemochromatosis be it Idiopathic or Secondary can cause congestive heart failure, arrhythmias, or a combination of both of these problems resulting in significant morbidities to the individual and frequently leading to mortalities.

OTHER ABNORMALITIES

OTHER INFILTRATING CONDITIONS THAT CAUSE MYOCARDIAL DISEASE

In addition to iron, there are other conditions that affect the heart by infiltrating the muscles of the heart such as:

1. Amyloidosis
2. Sarcoidosis
3. Leukemia
4. Loefflers

These conditions can individually affect the heart by infiltration because of the abnormal cells and/or substances that they produce. The result can also be congestive heart failures and other cardiac arrhythmias.

What must be kept in mind in outlining the above mentioned problems is that frequently when an individual presents with heart failure and cardiac arrhythmias and none of the usual diagnosis can be said to be the cause of the patient's problems, by the process of elimination, then it is important that one start thinking about some of these conditions just outlined above.

OTHER TYPES OF HEART DISEASE

VALVULAR HEART DISEASE

One category of congenital heart disease associated with disease of the valves is

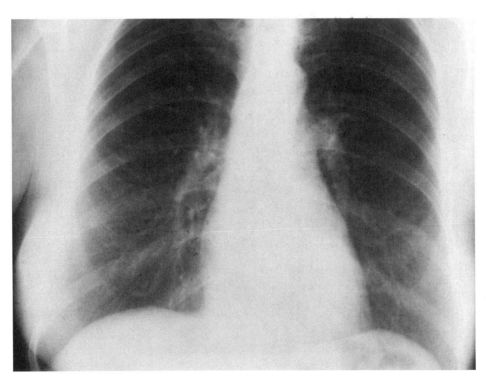

Figure 4.8. A normal chest x-ray.

called valvular heart disease. The heart has three separate valves; the mitral valve, the aortic valve, and the tricuspid valve. Each one of these valves can become narrowed causing what is called mitral stenosis, aortic stenosis, tricuspid stenosis. By the same token, one may also have what is called regurgitation of the mitral valve, regurgitation of the aortic valve, or regurgitation of the tricuspid valve. The leaflet of the valve, when damaged, becomes incompetent. Therefore, blood regurgitates back toward the valve causing problems in the overall function of the valve.

CONGENITAL HEART DISEASE

Valvular heart diseases can be experienced in all age groups (infancy to old age).

In infants and young children, they are due to congenital valvular heart disease. There are other conditions associated with congenital heart disease than cause illness at an early age, causing a baby to be very sick, where they have different chambers of the heart that are damaged. Also, there may be different holes in the heart that do not belong there and need to be closed otherwise, the child will not grow properly and will be sick all the time.

RHEUMATIC HEART DISEASE

In adults, valvular heart diseases are most likely due to rheumatic heart disease associated with infection of the valve. This can be caused by a strep organism. Group A

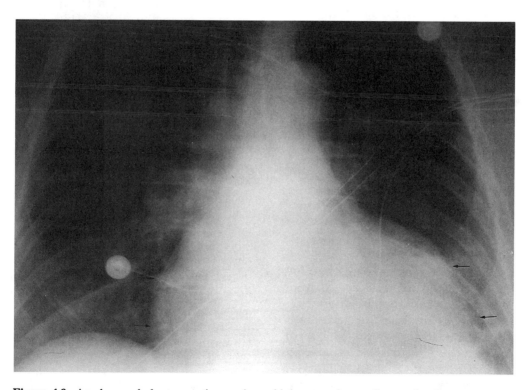

Figure 4.9. An abnormal chest x-ray in a patient with hypertensive cardiovascular disease showing heart failure as a result of chronic hypertension with secondary coronary artery disease leading to an enlarged heart and heart failure with arrows showing enlarged bother of right heart and arrows showing enlarged bother of left heart with pleural effusion. (fluid in lower left lung)

Streptococci can cause rheumatic heart disease leading to mitral valve stenosis because of the damage to the valve by the infection, which leads to a spectrum of diseases. These can start from mitral valve stenosis, all the way to mitral regurgitation. It is almost immediately apparent that if one has had rheumatic fever, the heart valve has been damaged. But, the person may have had rheumatic fever and had not known it because it was somewhat subclinical. Later on in life, he/she may develop a resulting heart condition. When the heart is properly evaluated, it may be discovered that there is a condition present indicating rheumatic heart disease. There may be heart failure and a rhythm abnormality of the heart (arrhythmias) all as a result of unknown previous heart damage associated with rheumatic fever. Also, the aortic valve and the tricuspid valve can be damaged by infection.

STENOSIS OF THE HEART VALVES

When one gets to be elderly, stenosis of the heart valves can be due to calcium deposits in the valves of the heart. This is associated with the aging process leading to first stenosis and then regurgitation of the valves of the heart.

COCAINE AND HEART DISEASE

Another form of heart disease that is, again, affecting the black community is the heart disease associated with the use of cocaine. It has now been discovered that sudden death can result from cocaine use due to heart failure. One can develop an acute abnormal rhythm of the heart from the use of cocaine. Cocaine use can result in a spasm that causes temporary occlusion of the coronary arteries, preventing blood and oxygen passage to the myocardium of the heart leading to a heart attack.

There is a whole host of cardiac abnormalities that can happen to the heart, and which lead to death, as a result of the use of cocaine. So, heroin and cocaine and crack addictions are devastating the black community resulting in psycho-social problems, an increase in crime, etc., but in terms of heart problems, cocaine and heroin are the two prevalent conditions in the black community causing the vast majority of drug-addiction associated heart diseases.

ALCOHOL AND HEART DISEASE

Another form of heart disease that is also prevalent in the African-American community is alcohol associated heart disease. Alcohol affects every organ in the human body. The myocardium (the muscle of the heart) becomes enlarged due to the effect of alcohol leading to alcohol induced cardiomyopathy. An increase in the incidence of coronary artery disease can evolve from the effect of alcohol. Alcohol causes an increase in the elevation of the blood pressure which in turn can cause an increased evidence of plaque deposition in the coronary arteries. This all can lead to heart attacks. So, alcohol abuse, (which affects 25% of the Black population of the United States) compares to only 12% of the general population being alcoholic. This disproportionate percentage of Black alcoholics is disturbing. Again, alcoholism is associated with stress, poverty, bigotry, and all the other negatives that one can think of that are associated with racism. An individual drinks to try to ease the pain of poverty and alcohol is inexpensive and one does not need a prescription for it. Yet, people do not understand that alcohol is a drug, and when taken in excess, can and does kill. I will speak later on about the effect of alcohol on the rest of the body in the chapter on alcoholism.

SUMMATION

In summary then, heart disease is disproportionately increased in the Black community as opposed to the white community. The root causes of this can be found in the effect of racism and bigotry leading to poverty and poor living conditions, poor diet and poor general health habits. All of these conditions are indirectly causing the increase in coronary artery disease and death in the Black community in a disproportionate percentage.

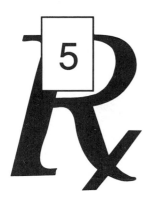

CANCER IN BLACKS IN THE UNITED STATES OF AMERICA

5

CHAPTER OUTLINE

THE INCIDENCE OF CANCER IN BLACKS IN THE UNITED STATES OF AMERICA

Next to heart disease, cancer is the leading cause of death in both men and women in this country. According to the American Cancer Society statistics, 1 million 100 thousand new cancer cases are expected to be diagnosed in 1991. Of that number, 545,000 new cases of cancer are expected to be diagnosed in men from all sites. 555,000 new cases of cancer are expected to be diagnosed in women from all sites. 514,000 people are expected to die in 1991 from cancer, 272,000 men and 242,000 women. There appears to be an increase in both the incidence of cancer and the death rate associated with cancer.

It is estimated that 161,000 cases of lung cancer will occur in the United States in 1991. Of this number, 101,000 cases in men and 60,000 cases in women. The estimated incidence of deaths from lung cancer in 1991 will be 143,000. Of that number, there will be 92,000 cases in men and 51,000 cases in women.

However, the predominant cancer in women is breast cancer. It is estimated that 175,900 cases of breast cancer will occur in 1991. 175,000 cases in women and 900 in men. Of this number, 44,800 will die; 300 cases in men and 44,500 in women. Although breast cancer is the predominant cancer in women, more women still die of cancer of the lung than cancer of the breast. In 1991, it is estimated that 51,000 women will die of cancer of the lungs as compared to 44,500 deaths from cancer of the breast. The reason for the higher incidence of lung cancer deaths in women is because the incidence of smoking has increased in women in the last 30 years.

In the same vein, statistics show that while more women have breast cancer, the estimated death from different cancers in the United States is that 18% of women will die of breast cancer, while 21% of women will

Table 1. The incidence of cancer from different sites in 1989 was:

Men		Women	
		Breast	28%
Colon and Rectum	14%	Colon and Rectum	15%
Leukemia and		Leukemia and	
Lymphomas	8%	Lymphomas	7%
Lung	20%	Lung	11%
Oral	4%	Oral	2%
Pancreas	3%	Pancreas	3%
Prostate	21%	Ovary	4%
Skin	3%	Skin	3%
Urinary	10%	Urinary	4%
		Uterus	9%
All Other	17%	All Other	14%[1]

1. Source: *American Cancer Society Statistics 1989*

die of lung cancer. In men, 35% will die of lung cancer, and 11% will die of colorectal cancer. And, 13% of women will die of colorectal cancer. Note that the incidences of death in colon cancer in women has also increased as compared to men.

The disturbing fact is that at presentation with all these different cancers in Blacks in the U.S., the cancer is almost always found to be more advanced. For instance, in cancer of the lung, 33% of Whites present with localized cancer of the lung as compared to only 27% of U.S. Blacks. But, there is a 6% difference in favor of the White individual being cured of localized cancer as compared to the Black person.

At presentation (according to the 1984 five-year survival statistics by the American Cancer Society) in all stages of cancer, 13% of Whites have a 5-year better survival chance as opposed to 11% of American Blacks. Again, note that this statistic mitigates in favor of the white population as compared to the African-American population.

In the case of colorectal cancer, 85% of Whites will present with a localized lesion, whereas only 76% of Blacks in the U.S. will present with the same. This is a difference of

9 percentage points between the white population and the black population in the U.S. Yet, in all stages of cancer of the colon and rectum as it relates to 5-year survival (regardless of the stage of cancer) there is a 53% chance of better 5-year survival in Whites. The American Black has only a 46% 5-year survival chance dealing with the stages of colorectal cancer. This is a 7 percentage point difference in a 5-year survival prognosis for the Black Americans as compared to the favored Whites.

In dealing with cancer of the breast; 90% of the white females have a better 5-year survival chance when they present with a localized lesion as compared to 86% of the Black females. In terms of all stages of breast cancer, 75% of the white females have a better 5-year survival chance, regardless of the stage of the cancer, as compared to 63% of black females. Again, this is a 12 percentage point difference in favor of the white female as compared to the Black female.

Another significant cancer that afflicts women is cancer of the cervix. Eighty-eight percent of white females present with localized lesions as compared to 84% of African-American females. In all stages, as it relates to a 5-year survival chance, 67% of white females have a better survival chance as compared to 59% of Black females.

In cancer of the ovary, as it relates to 5-year survival, 83% of white females have localized lesions and 79% Black females. In all stages, however, the difference isn't that much, 37% 5-year survival of all stages of ovarian cancer as opposed to 36% in Black females. The reason for this is because cancer of the ovary is such a devastating cancer, and almost always, cancer of the ovary, when discovered, is discovered in a fairly advanced stage. There are many variables as to why this is so, mostly the failure to perform a pelvic sonogram at an early point in evaluation of women is responsible. If one does a sono-

gram of the ovary as part of a routine yearly evaluation, it is probable that a large number of cancers of the ovary will be detected early. If one depends only on palpitation, one is likely to miss the cancer of the ovary and not detect it at an early stage.

Also, uterine cancer is a significant cancer in women. Ninety-one percent of white females who present with a localized lesion have a better 5-year survival chance as compared to 71% Black females. This is a significant 20 percentage difference. In terms of all stages of cancer taken together, 83% of white females have a better 5-year survival chance as compared to 53% of Black females. This is a 30 percentage point difference. White females when experiencing discomfort and unexplained vaginal bleeding are more likely to go to the doctor sooner to seek attention and get the appropriate Pap test performed. This will determine if there is uterine cancer which can lead to a D&C to detect uterine endometrial tissue to make a diagnosis. Therefore, appropriate treatment can be given sooner because the cancer has been found at an earlier stage. Black females tend to procrastinate because when they are spotting, they think that there is nothing seriously wrong, or they do not have the money to pay the doctor. Or, they wait because they don't have the time because they are busy working or have a house full of children—so they neglect themselves. Therefore, when they present to the clinic (where most Black women receive their medical care) the clinic may not be well-equipped to take care of them. Also, the health professionals that take care of them oftentimes are not experienced enough to take care of this problem. Probably it is because of a combination of these factors that there is a 30 percentage difference in the 5-year survival rate in favor of the white women over African-American women.

CANCER OF THE BLADDER

In cancer of the bladder, 88% of white women have a better 5-year survival chance as apposed to 80% of Black American females. All stages taken together, 77% of Whites have a better 5-year survival in bladder cancer as compared to 56% of Blacks in the U.S. Again, there is a 24% difference. The reason for this is usually the lack of understanding of one's body. If one has to urinate frequently and has pressure in the lower abdomen, many people don't understand what this means. If someone is seeing blood in the urine, there is a tendency to rely on self-diagnosis as opposed to going to the doctor for a urinalysis (to see if there are red cells in it which represents microhematuria). This can lead to a quick in-office evaluation. Most urologists are equipped to do a sonogram and IVP in the office and a renal scan. If a cystoscopy can be performed at a very early stage of this disease and appropriate diagnosis can be made, treatment can be rendered rather quickly to help these individuals survive. However, if one does not go to the doctor, or to the appropriate sub-specialist for these tests, one is doomed to an early death from cancer of the bladder and/or other types of cancer.

CANCER OF THE PROSTATE GLAND

Eighty-five percent of white males have the chance of a localized prostate cancer and an 88% better 5-year survival as opposed to 70% of Black American males having a 79% 5-year survival rate and having a localized lesion. If the lesion is localized, this implies that it is in an early stage and can be removed so that one can be cured. This is really essential in all types of cancers because once the cancer reaches the next stage, it becomes more difficult to cure. So, regardless of the type of cancer, one needs to discover the cancer at its earliest possible stage in order to try and cure it.

Seventy-two percent in all stages of cancer of the prostate in white men have a 72% 5-year survival as compared to 60% 5-year survival in the Black American male. The reason for this is that cancer of the prostate is a very difficult cancer to treat. It metastasizes very quickly to the bone, and the lung. It causes tremendous pain and early death, and if detected too late, one is doomed.

WHAT IS CANCER?

Cancer is when a cell, one single cell in the body, becomes defective. The word defective, here, means that the cell loses its contact inhibition. Contact inhibition is, for instance, if one takes a growing cell and places it in a petri dish, once the cell hits a surface, it loses the ability to stop growing. When the cell hits a particular surface, this is supposed to inhibit the cell from growing, and if the cell is not capable of doing this, it loses its contact inhibition and grows abnormally. The cell grows too fast, and its growing is uncontrolled and unorganized. This cell multiplies into hundreds, thousands and eventually millions of cells, and this becomes a cancerous growth. In order for a cell to grow, a cell must, by definition, use protein, amino acid, and other substances produced by the human body. Naturally, the cancer is using these substances to grow. This is one reason why the person becomes weak and loses weight. The person is in conflict with the cancerous growth which is using the proteins and the different substances needed by the body to grow. Also, it is growing in an uncontrolled fashion. Normal cell growth is based on biological law so that they only grow when it is time, and necessary to replace other cells that have died. These cells use the exact amount of substances that they need to grow. When the time comes for them to stop growing, they stop. But, cancer cells have no law or rule of growth. It is haphazard growth in an uncontrolled fashion (cancerous growth). The cancerous growth can either grow locally in the beginning, or it can find its way into the lymphatic system. In order for cancer to grow from one spot to the next, it must first enter into the blood stream, and then pass into the lymphatic system. But, it has to circulate in the body, into the lymphatic system. And then, from there it grows. Even if the lymph node is right next to it, it doesn't grow unless it has circulated in the body before passing into the lymphatic system. Unfortunately, this is what makes metastases so difficult to evaluate. The eye cannot see it, one can't put the entire body under a microscope to see if there are metastatic sites. The cell has to grow large enough so that it can become visible (through x-ray) so that it can be detected. Then, one can make a diagnosis whether or not the cancer has spread.

CANCER PROMOTERS

The biology of cancer is very complicated, and very complex. Today, it is believed that in the natural state, individuals are somewhat scheduled to have cancer because of heredity. This cancerous gene was probably transmitted to the fetus in utero as part of the genetic package that the fetus received from either the mother or father. After the end of embryonic growth, this particular cancerous gene gets turned off for some reason and remains dormant. The question is, what turns it on? It is believed that a number of things can stimulate this cancerous gene. It may be a virus which is cancer promoter. It may be a food substance that may be a cancer promoter. There are a whole host of cancer promoters and different types of carcinogens in the water and air. There are known carcinogens in the food that we eat and in the work place. Also, there are known carcinogens such as cigarettes.

Smoking definitely leads to cancer of the lung and cancer of the oropharynx. Those who snuff and chew tobacco are basically chewing a known carcinogen. Tobacco contains tar and this tar definitely is a carcinogen. If one were to shave the back of a laboratory animal (a mice or rat), paint that area with tar (examining the cells under a microscope before the tar was put on) and, let the tar remain there for a significant period of time, one will find that these cells have changed characteristics and are becoming cancerous. There is no room for argument here, because these are statements of fact.

Cigarettes reduce the average life span from 20–30 years. It is an addicting substance (nicotine) and, unfortunately, the incidence of smoking by Black Americans is very high, as is the incidence of drinking alcohol. The combination of cigarette smoking and alcohol drinking leads to a very high incidence of what is called head and neck cancer. Because alcohol irritates tissue, and anything that constantly irritates the tissue can lead to cellular changes, which can lead to cancer. Also, there is direct, undisputed evidence that the nicotine contained in cigarettes stimulates acid production and leads to a high incidence of ulcers of the stomach. Also, individuals who have emphysema and other chronic bronchitic conditions have a very high incidence of ulcers of the stomach. The fact is that the more one smokes, the sicker one is going to get, and the sooner one is going to die. There are no longer questions about it.

HOW DO CANCER PROMOTERS CAUSE CANCER?

It is believed that if one were "scheduled" to have cancer because of hereditary reasons, it is in the body lying dormant. If one takes a cancer promoter over a long period of time, it accumulates in the system and is going to stimulate the dormant gene. Then, the dormant gene manifests itself in a way that the cell loses its contact inhibition, and the cancer growth begins. An example of a cancer promoter, for instance, may be the red or yellow dyes in our food that are either outright carcinogens or are cancer promoters.

CANCER OF THE COLON

When one eats a lot of red meat, we need to digest it. In order to do this, we need to use a lot of bile salt made by the liver, which is carried by the gallbladder into the stomach to emulsify it. These bile salts are needed to digest the red meat, otherwise, it would sit there and not get digested.

In the process of digesting red meat, the stomach and colon are constantly being irritated by the excess bile salts. These bile salts are known to be an irritant to the lining of the colon. Anything that irritates in this fashion can cause abnormal cell proliferation. This can promote cancer. Therefore, there is usually a high incidence of cancer of the colon in individuals who have a diet high in red meat.

CONSTIPATION

When one becomes constipated it is because there is not enough bulky food or bran in the diet to promote regular bowel movements. This is dangerous because cancer promoters and carcinogens in the food stay in the colon too long. This exposes the tissues in the colon to carcinogens and cancer promoters, thereby resulting in cancer of the colon.

CANCER OF THE BREAST

Fat is needed in order for the body to have a strong biochemical skeletal system to build hormones. One needs this biochemical skeleton to be ingested. Even though the body makes its own fat, we need to take in fat from the outside in order to make a sufficient amount of hormones for the body to function properly.

However, if a woman takes in too much fat from eating red meat, she is exposing her breast tissue to too much stimulation from estrogen. Therefore, the more estrogen that one exposes breast tissue to, the more likely it is that one is going to develop breast cancer.

It is known that the more children a woman has, the less chance she has of developing breast cancer. The reason for this is because the breast tissue is given a break from the effect of estrogen because she is pregnant. The longer a woman is pregnant, the more rest the breast tissues receive. A woman who is going to develop breast cancer because of hereditary reasons can hasten the development by eating too much red meat, and by exposure to too much estrogen.

The birth control pill, though it has world wide importance in terms of the containment of the growth of the population (especially in poor countries) is dangerous. If one were to ask "is there an association between the birth control pill and the incidence of breast cancer?", the answer is "yes, most definitely". Multiple articles (paid for by the drug companies who are involved in making the birth control pills) would like us to believe otherwise. The fact is—birth control pills are very dangerous.

Birth control pills are very dangerous for a variety of other medical reasons. One of these reasons is the development of the so-called hypercoaguable state, which leads to phlebitis and clot formation in the leg, which in turn leads to pulmonary embolism, i.e. throwing a clot to your lungs. Individuals who take birth control pills have a lower level of antithrombin III. Antithrombin III is a substance that is needed for the native heparin that we secrete in our body to function properly. When there occurs a decrease in the antithrombin III one therefore has a predisposition to the development of clots. There is no question about it, birth control pills may cause these problems to occur.

Therefore, the thing to do is to avoid the pill at all costs if one can find some other means of contraception. One should contact her gynecologist and try to arrange this. Certainly, if one has a predisposing reason to worry about breast cancer, namely a sister had breast cancer, or mother had breast cancer, then taking the birth control pill is not advisable. Bear in mind, that 1 out of every 9 women in the United States is likely to have breast cancer during their lifetime.

In order to safeguard against breast cancer, a woman is advised to learn how to do a breast self-examination. If a lump is found in her breast, she is to go to the doctor immediately to have that lump evaluated, and, if necessary, a biopsy should be taken to try to diagnose the nature of the lump.

At the age 35, (for women who have high incidence of breast cancer in their family), it is recommended that a baseline mammogram be performed, and that the breasts be examined anywhere from 2–3 times per year. Also, one should learn how to do a careful breast examination at the appropriate time of the month, (around the menstrual period). If a woman has no incidence of breast cancer in her family, the age of 40 is the time (according to the American Cancer Society) for a baseline mammogram to be performed. This ought to be performed in conjunction with the breast examination. To do the mammogram alone, without having the breasts examined, is not effective. It is always good to get both examined because one doesn't have to have a palpable mass in the breast to have breast cancer. One may have other lesions that are associated in the nipple. If one sees a discharge coming from the nipple, this discharge ought to be evaluated by a physician promptly. And, it should be sent to Cytology to be examined under the microscope to see whether it's a cancerous

discharge or not. In addition, an unexplained discharge in a woman's breast needs medical attention because it could mean that there is some endocrine abnormality that is manifesting itself by galactorrhea, (milk in the breast at an unexpected time). If the discharge is bloody, the woman must go and have it checked. If she notices that the nipple is now becoming inverted and retracted, she has to have it evaluated. If she notices that she is having unexplained pain in the breast, she should go and have it evaluated. If the breast becomes swollen, she should have it evaluated because certain breast cancers manifest themselves by the swelling of the breast and discoloration, such as redness. Any type of abnormality noticed in the breast, that is different from the norm, should be evaluated as soon as possible.

For women at age 50, it is recommended that they have a yearly mammogram. The radiation that is emitted when one has a mammogram performed is far less of a problem than allowing one's self to develop breast cancer.

Also, somewhere between 20–30% of women who have breast cancer have cysts in the breasts, (fibrocystic disease of the breast). These are not precancerous lesions, but, because 20–30% of women who have breast cancer also have had cysts in the breasts, it makes one worry about any lump in the breast. Therefore, women with fibrocystic disease of the breasts, when they reach the age of 35, should have the breasts examined frequently.

BREAST EXAMINATION

A breast examination is a procedure that is learned by an oncologist. There are certain gynecologists who probably know how to do a very good exam. However, be careful to have a thorough breast examination. It is very important for the doctor to palpate under the axilla, under the arm, to look for nodes because sometimes one may not feel a lump in the breast at all, but may feel the lump under the arms. And, this could indicate breast cancer. The reason why it is important to sample the nodes under the arm is because even if one node is positive, it has statistical meaning as to the prognosis of the woman who has this breast cancer. One positive node means one thing, 4 positive nodes means another, and negative nodes also mean something quite different.

There is a technique on how to examine the breasts. The arms are to be extended in front of her so that one looks at the symmetry of the breasts to see if there is any retraction of the skin. Then, put the hand underneath the arms and palpate carefully for nodes. Then, the woman has to have one arm down and lie flat on her back, with one arm underneath her head, and one of the breasts has to be evaluated very carefully. Then, the arm is put *down*, the other arm again is put under the head, and the other breast is examined for abnormalities. This is a delicate type of examination and it ought to be done very carefully by a physician who has experience in how to properly examine women's breasts.

WHAT TO DO WHEN A LUMP IS DISCOVERED IN YOUR BREAST?

When a lump is discovered in the breast, the first step is to have a mammogram. However, it may not be very effective to do a mammogram on an 18 year old woman because the breast tissue is too solid and not very much will appear on the mammogram. But, between the ages of 25 and upward, it is possible to get a good mammogram. The purpose of the mammogram is to evaluate the anatomy of the breast to see if there are calcifications, because some calcifications can have malignant characteristics to them, and some calcifications can be benign. It is important to also realize that one may have to perform a needle localization of a certain type of calcifications before one can tell whether they are benign or malignant. This is also necessary to determine the characteristics of the lump in question. Sometimes, the lump may be palpated by the physician; yet, it is not picked up by the mammogram and it could be a cancerous lump. So, it's important that both a mammogram and examination are performed.

The next step is to be evaluated by a surgeon who will decide to do a biopsy, or a needle aspiration, and to send the material for pathological evaluation.

After this, if the tissue is a cyst, breathe easy. If it comes back that it is cancerous, then, a decision has to be made on the type of surgical procedure needed to be performed. The choices are: a lumpectomy, a lumpectomy with axillary dissection, or a modified radical mastectomy.

LUMPECTOMY

If a woman decides to have a lumpectomy done, it is important that the implications of a lumpectomy are fully explained to her. If she has decided definitely on the lumpectomy, then she should be aware that a lumpectomy without nodal dissection could mean that metastatic disease to the nodes could be present without her knowing about it. It is preferable to do a lumpectomy with axillary node dissection. After breast tissue is taken out, it will be decided, based on the location of the tumor, the degree of invasion of the tumor into the muscle, the size of the tumor (1 cm. to 4 cm.), whether the tumor estrogen and the progesterone receptors are negative or positive, and whether the nodes under the axillary are either positive or negative. At this point, following appropriate laboratory tests and x-ray studies, then the tumor can be staged.

Prior to breast surgery, it is important to have a chest x-ray and a complete blood count and complete blood chemistries done.

Even if the chemistries are completely normal, one may still have cancer in the liver. It is not at all unusual to have documented metastases to the liver and have a blood chemistry that is completely normal. So, having normal blood chemistries is not enough to determine that the woman has no metastases to the liver. One has to perform either the abdominal ultrasound or an abdominal CAT scan with views of the liver to determine metastases. Because breast cancer metastasizes to the bone very rapidly and easily, it is important to have a bone scan done. If one has liver metastases, and bone metastases, do not try to perform a radical mastectomy. One cannot help the woman out if she already has metastatic disease to her bone, liver, or other places. At this point, examine the tissue to establish a diagnosis. Also, if the lump can be removed, remove the tumor by removing the lump. This is beneficial because it also allows one to have tissue for estrogen and progesterone receptor studies. This is very important because these are used to determine the possible behavior of the tumor, namely the response of the tumor to treatment. Receptor positive tumors respond better to chemotherapy as compared to receptor negative tumors. Receptive positive tumors allow the physician to be able to offer the patient Tamoxifen treatment (hormonal manipulation treatment using Tamoxifen).

The menstrual status of the woman is very important to determine—because premenopausal women have one set of response to treatment as compared to postmenopausal women. Taking tissue allows one to be able to do DNA studies via flow cytometry to determine whether the tumor is anaploid or has diploid cells. Women who are premenopausal respond to chemotherapy better than women who are postmenopausal.

Women who are postmenopausal and who have receptor positive, benefit much more from 3–5 years of hormonal treatment with Tamoxifen (as opposed to women who are premenopausal and women who are receptor negative). Both women who are postmenopausal and are ER positive and postmenopausal who are ER negative can be treated with combination chemotherapy.

Based on the latest recommendations (published in 1988 by the National Cancer Institute), women who have stage I disease (receptor negative or receptor positive) benefit a great deal in terms of 5-year survival chance after receiving 6 months of combination chemotherapy with either Cytoxan, Adriamycin and 5 FU or Cytoxan, Methotrexate and 5 FU.

If the woman has no bone metastases and no liver metastases, however, she does have a node positive tumor (even one node) a combination chemotherapy is needed. The most sensitive combination chemotherapy available is Cytoxan, Adiamycin and 5 FU to treat the woman who has nodes positive, regardless of the receptor status of the tumor. If the woman is receptor positive, her chances of response is documented to be higher when taken in aggregates to chemotherapy.

RADIOTHERAPY

Radiotherapy still plays a role in cancer treatment based on the size of the tumor, and the choice of the patient. If the patient does not want to receive chemotherapy and has a Stage 1 lesion, (2 cm.) she may choose to receive radiotherapy to the breast at the appropriate time (when the wound is well healed). Bear in mind that she is only being treated locally with radiotherapy and there is no provision for distant micrometastases. Hence, there is an advantage of combination chemotherapy to radiotherapy. If one chooses to be treated by both radiotherapy and chemotherapy, one has to keep in mind that she is also being exposed to a high incidence of a second malignancy that is known to occur secondary to cytotoxic agents. The more the cytoxic agent, the more likely that within 7–10 years a second malignancy (such as chronic myelogenous leukemia) might develop in the patient. Also, other types of malignancies may develop as manifestations of cytotoxic agents. It is important that the patient is well advised and gives an informed consent. So, when she is receiving these treatments, she is fully aware of the type of treatment being administered. If the type of treatment that she receives is based on the doctor's understanding of the problem, it is important to make the patient and the family aware that there is a chance of the development of a secondary malignancy within 7–10 years.

Systemic chemotherapy is frequently associated with amenorrhea. The patient may develop the inability to menstruate while receiving cytotoxic agents. It is recommended that a woman not become pregnant when she is receiving cytotoxic agents because the baby may be affected adversely by the side effects of the cytotoxic agents.

TAMOXIFEN

Tamoxifen is a medication that is used in women who are receptor positive. This medication has certain side effects. These include: hypercalcemia, (high serum calcium,) and also some women have menopausal type symptoms, such as irritation and hot flashes. It is otherwise tolerated, and one has to follow the woman with a serum calcium for several months after the medication is started, and then every 2–3 months thereafter. Also, a complete blood count to monitor the woman should be prescribed.

As for the side effects of the cytotoxic agents mentioned above, Adriamycin has a bone marrow toxicity. It can lower the white count, the platelet count, and the red cell count. It can also affect the heart causing cardiac abnormalities. Before the medication

is started, a rest MUGA ought to be performed to have a baseline for the ejection fraction. This is a sensitive way of determining the cardiac output. Every 2–3 months during treatment, another rest MUGA ought to be performed to make sure that the ejection fraction is not decreasing because this could be an indication of cardiac toxicity. It is also important to have a baseline EKG performed to be sure of what one is starting out with.

Cytoxan can cause loss of hair, and Cytotoxin can also cause bladder problems with cystitis. Check the urine frequently to see if there are red cells which could be an indication of Cytoxan toxicity to the bladder. It can also cause bone marrow toxicity such as a lowered white count, lowered platelet count, and lowered red cell count.

As for 5 fluorouracil, this again causes bone marrow toxicity and can cause lowered white counts, lowered platelets, and lowered red cell count. It can also be associated with mucositis (sores of the mouth). The patient ought to be informed and prophylactically treated with either Nystatin or Mycelex troche to prevent the development of mucositis. In some patients, there is a darkening of the skin of the back of the hand that is associated with 5 FU. This also should be outlined to the patient before starting treatment.

MEN WITH BREAST CANCER

It is also important to mention that men with breast cancer are also treated the same way. Everything stated above as it relates to treatment for women with breast cancer also applies to men. The approach is just about the same. It is estimated that in 1991, 900 men will develop cancer of the breast and 300 of these men will die of breast cancer. In fact, breast cancer in men can at times be an extremely accelerated malignant disease with fulminant complications.

PSYCHOLOGICAL STRESS AND BREAST CANCER

Women who have breast cancer are under tremendous psychological stress and need not only professional support from the physician, and nurses, but she also needs understanding from her family. The American Cancer Society has all kinds of programs. "I Can Cope" and "Reach to Recovery" type of programs can help women through this difficult period. Women should contact their local American Cancer Society for assistance so they can join these different programs to learn more about breast cancer. It is especially important so that they can cope during the period of chemotherapy and recovery. There are all sorts of published pamphlets that deal with these issues, and also different prostheses the women need to use for the missing part of the breast. Different local American Cancer Societies will be more than happy to work with these women to try to help them cope with this very difficult disease.

ADVANCED STAGE CANCER

How does one deal with the women (or men) who have cancer in an advanced stage such as bony mets and liver mets and stage 4 cancer? They oftentimes suffer from a lot of pain, and the inability to eat, because they have become weakened by the cancer. It is important to sustain them with pain medications, and continue to give them palliative chemotherapy, in order to try to retard the progression of the cancer. It is also important to sometimes try ablative medical adrenalectomy to try to arrest the growth and progress of the tumor. Appropriate measures with replacement of corticosteroids and different steroids ought to be instituted to treat the adrenal insufficiency that is being induced. Oftentimes, this is a last resort that one uses in order to try to buy a few more months for these patients who are in this very advanced stage of the disease.

HOSPICE

Hospice and the whole hospice concept is very important in this day and age. Individuals can benefit greatly from the removing of stress from the family unit by joining Hospice. Also, home therapy with IV fluids, and around the clock analgesics, are variables that ought to be used in the handling and treating patients in the advanced stages of the tumor.

BREAST CANCER SUMMARY

In summary, breast cancer is a treatable disease if found in Stage I or Stage II, and even with one or two nodes positive in the Stage II lesion. There is a significant incidence of 5-year survival chance in these women. The important thing to understand is that early detection is the most important aspect in breast cancer. For the Black females to try to reverse the trend of presenting to the doctor with an advanced stage disease, early detection is essential. Again, the white female has a 90% 5-year survival chance, and a 90% chance of presenting with a localized lesion as opposed to 86% 5-year survival chance in the Black females. In all stages of breast cancer, the white female has a 75% 5-year survival chance, while this applies to only 63% of Black females. There is a 12 percentage point difference which is in favor of the white female. To reverse this trend, early detection techniques must be taught in the Black community. It is recommended that these women read more frequently all available materials concerning breast cancer. The clinics need to take it upon themselves to educate Black women and do a more thorough job of early detection of breast cancer. By teaching Black women how to perform breast self-exams, and the value of mammograms, (at age 35–40 if the woman is in a high risk group and at age 40 for any woman to have a baseline mammogram and at age 50 to have a yearly mammogram). Of course, their risk should decrease with frequent breast examinations by physicians who know how to examine breasts, which is very crucial because it is not safe for a woman to discover a lump in her breast and keep it to herself. Because, by the time she presents to the doctor it is often too late. However, if the tumor is found at a Stage 1 or 2, a woman has a potentially curable disease, as opposed to a treatable disease. If it is a Stage 3 or Stage 4, it is an incurable disease.

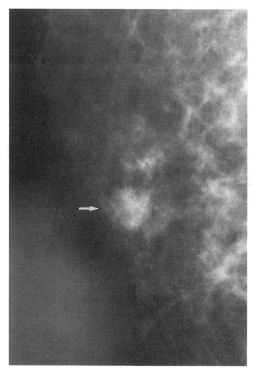

Figure 5.1. Mammogram showing 1 cm in diameter malignant mass in left breast. (arrow)

INCIDENCE OF CANCER
OF THE COLON

As the statistics published by the American Cancer Society state, 157,500 cases of cancer of the colon and rectum are expected to occur in 1991. 79,000 cases of colon and rectum cancer are expected to occur in men and 78,500 are expected to occur in females. 60,500 individuals are expected to die from colorectal cancer in 1991. 30,000 in men and 30,500 in women.

Cancer of the colon is characterized by a staging system, (Dukes' staging system). Dukes' A is basically when the tumor is confined to the colon, and Dukes' B is a tumor with extension into the pericolic fat and the serosa. Dukes' C is a tumor that has metastasized to the regional nodes, (mesenteric lymph nodes). Also, Dukes' D is a tumor with distant metastases such as to the bone, the lungs, and the liver.

BILE ACID AS A POSSIBLE
CANCER PROMOTER

The root causes of cancer of the colon and rectum vary a great deal. Genetics increase the chances of developing cancer of the colon or rectum. A family history increases the possibility about 50% greater than the general population. Certainly diet plays a role in the development of cancer of the colon. In particular a diet that is high in red meat and fat, can predispose one to this kind of cancer. The reason, as stated before, is that when someone eats red meat and other food (with a lot of fat in it) one has to use a lot of bile acids from the liver, into the gallbladder, and then into the stomach to digest the food. Because we need bile acids for fat to be digested, it leads to a lot of bile acid being transferred into the colon resulting in irritation. This bile acid is believed to cause irritability that leads to the promotion of cancer. Bile acids are considered to be cancer promoters.

CARCINOGENS AND
CANCER PROMOTERS

In addition, the foods we eat are often times associated with a lot of carcinogens such as, food coloring, preservatives, and seasonings, that are used to keep the food fresh or to season them.

If one had a dormant cancer gene in one's body, it requires some sort of a cancer promoter to stimulate it. Sometimes the cancer promoter could be a virus or other type of microorganism (such as fungus or a bacteria) or sometimes just food substances that one eats, can stimulate the gene and then lead to the development of cancer.

WHAT ARE THE SYMPTOMS OF COLON CANCER?

If one suddenly develops constipation, this could be a symptom of colon cancer. Unexplained diarrhea can also be a symptom of colon cancer. Cramping in the lower abdomen (that has no explanation) could be a symptom of colon cancer. Blood in the stool, bright red blood per rectum could be a symptom indicative of cancer of the colon. Unexplained weight loss, loss of appetite, and unexplained inguinal hernias can be a sign indicating the possibility of colon cancer, (if one develops a hernia without having been involved in heavy lifting or other activities that can lead to a hernia). Also, if one is constipated and there is a lesion in the colon that causes obstruction to the normal flow of stool, the constant straining that is involved in trying to move one's bowel can lead to the development of an inguinal hernia. So, unexplained inguinal hernia in an individual 35 and older can be first sign that this person is developing cancer of the colon. Therefore, if a patient develops an inguinal hernia (without any reasonable explanation), it is a good

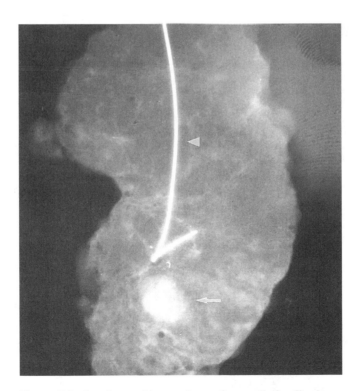

Figure 5.2. Specimen of breast tissue after needle localization. Malignant mass in breast. (arrow) Guide wire arrow head.

71

practice prior to treating that hernia surgically to evaluate the patient either via a colonoscopic exam and/or barium enema to look for the possibility of an obstructing colonic lesion. Naturally people can develop inguinal hernias for a variety of reasons, and yet don't have cancer of the colon, but because of the possibility of cancer, it is important to keep it in mind.

WHAT TO DO IF ONE SUSPECTS COLON CANCER

Go to the doctor. Explain what the symptoms are. Ask the appropriate questions. Have all the necessary blood tests, and have them interpreted properly, and then proceed to have a GI evaluation, either a colonoscopic exam or a barium enema. Sometimes both of them are necessary, depending on the circumstances. If these are normal, then at this point the doctor should proceed to have an evaluation of the upper GI tract to make sure that is not where the problem is originating. It is only then that one can rule out a GI malignancy because the bowel was evaluated, and the stomach was evaluated. Keep in mind that if one only has a barium enema, one is not evaluating the lower bowel properly because the last 25 cm. of the lower bowel is not evaluated by the barium enema. A significant percentage of cancer is found in this location.

For this reason it is important to do either the flexible sigmoidoscopic exam in conjunction with the barium enema, or the colonoscopic exam because the colonoscopic exam evaluates the entire bowel. If this is

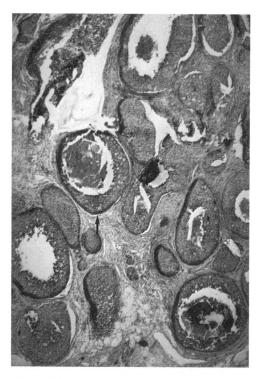

Figure 5.3. Intraductal Carcinoma of the breast. (arrow)

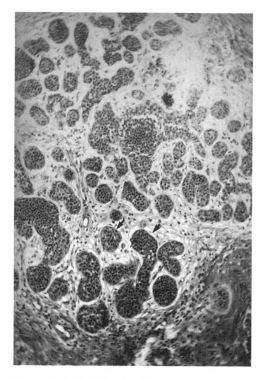

Figure 5.4. Lobular Carcinoma of the breast. (arrows)

normal, then the doctor should proceed to evaluate the upper GI tract, namely, the stomach and the small bowel because there are such things as cancer of the small bowel. This cannot be detected from the colonoscopic exam. This can only be detected (so far to this date) by an evaluation of the stomach with a small bowel follow through. So, if one suspects cancer, and it's not in the lower tract, then one has to evaluate the stomach and do a small bowel follow through because there are such things as lymphoma of the small bowel, cancer of the small bowel, in addition to cancer of the stomach. For that matter, the bleeding may be the result of ulcers. One doesn't need to have pain to have ulcers. One could bleed significantly to the point requiring a blood transfusion and still be thoroughly asymptomatic from the stomach. So, the GI tract needs to be evaluated from the esophagus all the way to the anus, and it is only when these things are found to be negative that one can be certain no GI pathology exists.

WHAT TO DO IF AN INDIVIDUAL HAS ANY OF THE ABOVE SYMPTOMS

The first thing to do is to go to a physician and have a thorough physical examination including a complete blood count, a serum ferritin, and the blood chemistries. Also, an examination of the stool for blood is crucial. Even if the patient's stool has no occult blood in it, the patient can still have cancer of the colon or the rectum because bleeding from this cancer is almost always intermittent. It takes around 15 ml. of blood intermixed with the stool to cause the hemoccult test performed to be positive. Because it

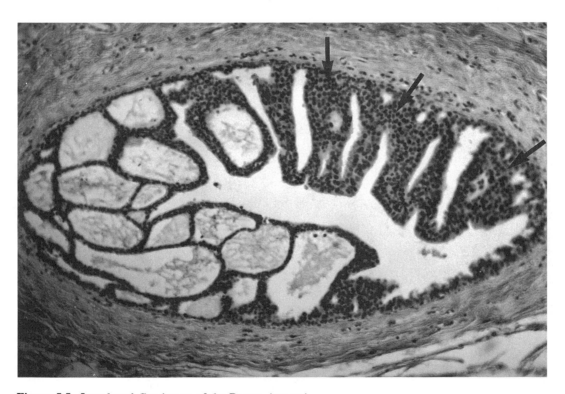

Figure 5.5. Intraductal Carcinoma of the Breast. (arrows)

is an intermittent process, further evaluation using a flexible sigmoidoscopic evaluation or colonoscopic evaluation should be performed. Coupled with this, a barium enema may be necessary based on the judgment of the physician. The serum ferritin is very important because it is the test that evaluates the total body iron store. One has to be very careful in how to interpret the serum ferritin because ferritin is a phase II reacting protein, and cancer is an inflammatory process. If there is a cancer present, it may falsely elevate the serum ferritin, it will not make it normal but it might obscure the upward range to make it seem as though it is normal. If the serum ferritin is normal, (10 through 125 or 100 to 300) it has to be understood that this is a range. If the physician sees a big husky guy who weighs 200 lbs. showing up in the office, who is 50 years old and is expected to have a serum ferritin of 250 and suddenly the serum ferritin is down to 50 or 40, even though this falls in the so-called "normal range", it is still an abnormal serum ferritin. It indicates that the patient is depleting his iron stores. It has to be understood that even though the hematocrit and the hemoglobin may be perfectly normal, the physician ought to evaluate the patient immediately for the possibility of cancer of the colon or of the stomach. Or, examine the patient for occult bleeding processes, (such as bleeding polyps or bleeding peptic ulcer) to explain why the serum ferritin is low. It is distinctly abnormal to be 200 lbs., 50 years old, and have a serum ferritin of 40 or 50. It

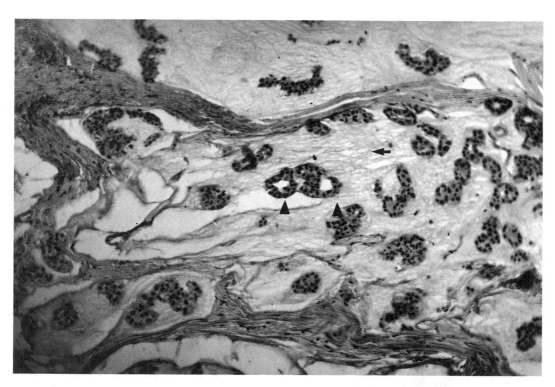

Figure 5.6. Mucus producing Carcinoma of the breast.
Mucus. (arrow)
Cancer cells. (arrow heads)

is crucial to take care of the problem immediately because at this stage one may be dealing with Dukes' A lesion, a lesion that is within the colon but has not yet invaded the serosa, or the fat of the area. If diagnosed soon enough, this patient may be cured.

RED CELL DISTRIBUTION WIDTH

Another test that is very important and can indicate early blood loss is the RDW (Red cell distribution width). Red cell distribution width, is used to do a complete blood count. This is very important because when the red cells are microcytic or macrocytic, it will cause the RDW to be elevated. So, the RDW is a more sensitive test than the scrum ferritin test in detecting the earliest indication that blood is being lost in the stool.

With this information, one may proceed to evaluate the patient for the possibility of iron loss as a result of chronic blood loss in the stool. Also, the RDW will be elevated if somebody is hemolyzing. The LDH (lactic dehydrogenase) will be high. If the RDW is elevated, pay attention to the first sign that blood is being lost in the stool because the patient's red cells have a different distribution to them. If the patient is losing blood occultly, it could mean that the patient is occultly bleeding from a lesion in the colon. So, try to detect the lesion early enough so that the patient may be cured. Because, by the time the patient has become anemic with low hemoglobin, low hematocrit and microcytosis, he/she has already lost the iron store (2 grams of iron) and has become microcytic (within 6–8 months). All the time the person

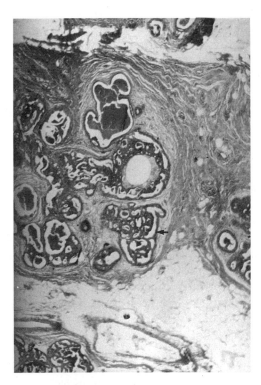

Figure 5.7. Intraductal Carcinoma of the breast. (arrow)

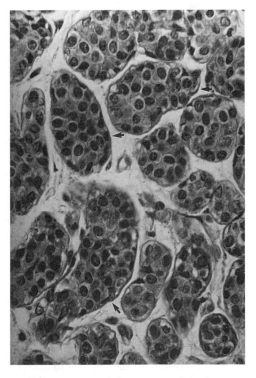

Figure 5.8. Lobular Carcinoma of the breast. (arrow)

75

has been bleeding, the cancer has been growing. By the time the patient presents with anemia, (which is now microcytic in nature) it is probably the result of blood loss secondary to the colon cancer. Also, they may already have a lesion (probably Dukes' B2 or C) which is advanced and has already metastasized (Dukes' D lesion). Now, it is already too late, and much more difficult to try to cure these individuals.

EVALUATION OF THE STOOL VIA THE HEMOCCULT TESTING

This is a very important thing to realize. The hemoccult evaluated blood found in the mouth all the way down to the anus. However, this test ought to be done properly. Because if it is not done properly, there can be false positives and false negatives.

FALSE POSITIVE STOOL HEMOCCULT TEST

False positives are associated with aspirin ingestion, and with arthritis medications such as non-steroidal anti-inflammatory medications. All these can cause this test to be falsely positive. Alka-seltzer will make it falsely positive because Alka-seltzer has aspirin in it. On the false negative side, one cannot take vitamin C. Vitamin C causes this test to become negative because it neutralizes the reaction. The chemical reaction that is involved in doing the hemoccult test is an oxidation reaction. However, Vitamin C is a reducing agent. So, when one takes Vitamin C and then has one's stool tested for occult blood, the chemical reaction will be neutralized, causing the test to be falsely negative. It is therefore very dangerous if you are in the cancer age group to be taking Vitamin C. Because, Vitamin C can, in fact, cause a physician to miss a cancer of the colon that you may be harboring if the physician did not warn you ahead of time not to take Vitamin

C for up to a week before you present to have your stool tested.

HOW DOES ONE APPROACH CANCER OF THE COLON IF IT IS DISCOVERED?

The Dukes' Staging System and Management of Colon Cancer

If one has cancer of the colon, and it is both adenocarcinoma and Dukes' A (it is within the colon and hasn't reached the serosa or the fat). This type of lesion is almost always surgically curable. Depending on the location of the cancer of the colon, the surgeon should be able to perform surgery and resect the colon, and the patient may not need a colostomy.

Almost always, a Dukes' A lesion does not require any further treatment after surgery. What is needed is that the patient is followed closely. And, the patient should have a colonoscopic exam done (6 months after surgery), (1 year after surgery), and then every year, thereafter. The patient should have this exam in addition to regular physical exams to be certain that there is no new cancer, or a recurrence of the same cancer.

If the patient is found to have a Dukes' B2 lesion, (a lesion that has involved the serosa and also the fat surrounding the colon in that area), this type of lesion should be surgically resected, and the patient should receive treatment with 5 Fluorouracil anywhere from 6 months to 1 year postop. The same procedure should be followed with colonoscopic exams (6 months), (1 year) and then (every year) thereafter. Again, this is to make sure that there is no recurrence. Also, the patient should be evaluated by complete blood counts and blood chemistries and stools for blood, (etc.).

If the patient is found to have a Dukes' C lesion, again, the lesion has to be resected and a sampling of nodes should be performed in the area to see if there is involvement of the mesenteric lymph nodes. If there is such involvement, the patient is staged as being a Dukes' C. Again, the patient, following re-section and the appropriate period of time (anywhere from 3–5 weeks postop), should receive 5 Fluorouracil with Leucovorin. Leu-covorin is a cancer modulator, immunomodu-lator, and it enhances the effect of the 5 FU. Again, this particular stage of cancer ought to be treated with 5 FU and Leucovorin, but the chances of curing these individuals are much less because of the involvement of the lymph nodes. But, close to 20–30% of pa-tients (based on statistics) can be cured using this technique.

An encouraging article was published (New England Journal of Medicine, Feb. 8, 1990, Volume 322) by Dr. Charles G. Mortel, regarding the use of Levamisole and Fluorouracil as adjuvant treatment for Dukes' C carcinoma of the colon. It was reported that there is an increased survival chance in patients who have Dukes' C cancer of the colon who were treated with Levamisole and Fluorouracil. Although more work needs to be done to confirm this report, the prelimi-nary data is very encouraging.

Stage Dukes' D lesion is when there are distant metastases to the liver, to the lungs, etc. It is not a curable stage of the dis-ease. Dukes' D cancer of the colon is not a curable lesion. Basically, it is treated with 5 FU for palliative reasons, and pain relief. These individuals are not likely to be cured of their colon cancer because of the ad-vanced metastases to the liver, the lung, etc.

The routine cancer marker that is being used for cancer of the colon and other GI malignancies is carcinoembryonic antigen (CEA). Unfortunately, it is not very specific because it is found to be elevated in a variety of conditions including: people who smoke heavily, have diabetes mellitus, and/or other types of cancer. However, if one discovers someone to have cancer of the colon or the stomach, it is helpful to have a baseline CEA. Then, as the treatment proceeds, moni-tor the treatment with the CEA. The CEA is valuable because although it is not a diagnos-tic test, it is a test that is used to monitor both the progress of the cancer, and the pro-gress of the treatment.

In summary then, both cancer of the colon and the rectum are curable diseases if detected at an early stage. The recommenda-tion is to present to the doctor at the first sign of weight loss, diarrhea, constipation (that is unexplained) and blood in the stool, etc. As soon as the doctor discovers unexplained low serum ferritin, it has to be evaluated.

A man can only lose blood normally through the GI tract. If one were to have a peculiar disease such as: paroxysmal noctur-nal hemoglobinuria, (PNH) where one loses iron in the urine. There is a rare condition in-volving the lungs where one can actually bleed into the lungs. And, there are instances where a man can lose blood in the urine from cancer of the bladder or the kidney. These conditions are easily perceivable be-cause of the presence of blood. The urine will be red. However, microscopic blood loss in the urine certainly is not sufficient to cause one to lose iron.

There are rare conditions that involve the colon that can cause one to lose blood and iron such as inflammatory bowel disease, (colitis) and Crohn's disease. These are also associated with blood loss chronically, and they can also cause one to become iron defi-cient. Inflammatory bowel disease is also as-sociated with an increased incidence of cancer of the colon. Once a male is in the cancer age group, and becomes iron defi-cient, cancer has to be considered by the physician. But, one can have cancer of the colon without being in the cancer age group, for instance, familial polyposis has increasing incidences of cancer of the colon and can definitely occur at an age much earlier.

EVALUATING FOR CANCER
OF THE COLON

Serum iron and total iron binding capacity (TIBC) are very inaccurate tests as a means of evaluating for cancer of the colon. They can be falsely elevated by so many different variables that it is not advisable to depend solely on them (serum iron and TIBC) to arrive at a diagnosis of iron deficient anemia. The most accurate test is a bone marrow aspiration, but this is an invasive procedure with some discomfort. It's not always necessary to have a bone marrow aspiration to make a diagnosis, however, in clinical practice (particularly in the hospital), frequently the hematologist will do the bone marrow because it is the most accurate way of evaluating the iron storage and iron deficiency. This lead to a GI workup that should lead to the correct diagnosis. But, with the serum ferritin being available, it is not always necessary to resort to a bone marrow to diagnose iron deficiency anemia. However, if one is anemic and it is not clear why, then bone marrow is the most accurate way to completely evaluate the anemia.

Women who are menstruating lose iron every month through the menstrual blood loss. So therefore, the number one disease of women in the world is iron deficiency anemia. At what point does one begin to consider cancer in a women who is iron deficient? Well, based on symptoms, if the woman is having rectal blood loss or if the woman is losing a lot of weight and having diarrhea and constipation. Usually, when a woman presents at age 40, and has iron deficiency that is when one has to be careful not to assume that the blood loss is only due to menstrual blood loss, because, age 35–40 falls into the cancer group. At this point, one needs to be very careful not to begin to treat the patient with iron therapy thinking that the iron deficiency is due only to menstrual blood loss. It may frequently be due to a combination of menstrual blood loss plus GI blood loss. So, at

age 40 a GI workup in a woman who has a low serum ferritin or who has absent iron store in the bone marrow ought to have a GI workup involving the lower bowel. If that is normal, evaluate the stomach and the small bowel to make sure that there is no cancer or other pathology associated with blood loss such as bleeding polyps or bleeding ulcers that can cause the iron blood loss. It is very dangerous to begin to treat women age 40 for iron deficiency anemia without a GI evaluation. Women lose blood through menstrual blood loss, and most women in this country are on a diet of one form or another. If they have had children, quite a bit of blood is lost during each delivery. This blood loss is often never replaced. If they were taking iron when they were carrying the baby, once they deliver the baby, they no longer continue to take iron and then they continue to menstruate and lose more iron that way. Women are often times on diets to prevent weight gain. These diets are always deficient in iron. This leads to the iron deficiency problem. So, the number one disease in women in the world is really iron deficiency. In the vast majority of women, African-American women in particular, because they are forced to survive on such a low income, eating food that is less rich in iron and different vitamins, are even more prone to iron deficiency anemia. Still, they ought to be evaluated properly before one begins to assume that all the blood is lost from menses and not from other GI pathology.

MORE ADVANCED STAGES OF
COLON CANCER IN BLACKS

As far as cancer of the colon is concerned, again it's the same thing. Almost always Black men and Black women present with a disease that is in an advanced stage. Again, for the same reasons, they do not go to the doctor very often and if they do go to the doctor, sometimes, they go to an inexperienced or unqualified doctor. They go to a clinic that is not very well equipped to take good care of them, or they don't go at all. As a result of this, they almost always present with a disease that is more advanced as compared to their white counterparts.

As evidenced by the statistics published by the American Cancer Society in 1984, whereby Whites had an 85% 5-year survival chance of localized lesions, and for Blacks it was a 76% 5-year survival chance when the lesion was localized they present only 76% of the time with localized lesion. This is a 9 percentage point which is quite significant.

COLORECTAL CANCER

As for all stages of colorectal cancer, the 5-year survival chance for Whites was 53%, and for Blacks it was 46%. Again, it is a significant difference in 5-year survival chances in all stages.

HEMORRHOIDS AS A SIGN OF COLORECTAL CANCER

If suddenly someone begins to suffer with hemorrhoids, it could be the first sign of cancer in the colon because the obstructing lesion is forcing the individual to strain at stooling. This leads to the development of hemorrhoids. If one has a new set of hemorrhoids that develop when in the cancer age group (35–40 onward), this could be the first presentation that there is cancer of the colon. In the process of evaluation these types of hemorrhoids, it is important to use a flexible sigmoidoscopy. Also, it may be necessary to do a colonoscopic examination to evaluate why suddenly the hemorrhoids may be causing pain, discomfort, and are bleeding. Hemorrhoids are not just always a result of being constipated. Sometimes, the constipation is due to an obstruction because of a mass or a polyp causing strain. The evaluation of hemorrhoids (suddenly developed) calls reasonably frequently for a lower GI evaluation. It is important to note that such an individual may have more

than just hemorrhoids. Statistics (published by the American Cancer Society) show that in 1991, 157,500 individuals will develop cancer of the colon and the rectum. And, some 60,500 of these individuals will die of this disease. But, keep in mind that the rest (those who don't die from this disease) are being cured by surgical resections, early detection, and by chemotherapy. So, cancer of the colon and rectum are definitely curable cancers if diagnosed early. The recommendation for early detection and treatment, and cure, is to know one's body. If one notices something different about one's bowel habits, go and seek medical care. There is no part of the anatomy that is sacred.

RECTAL EXAMINATION

A rectal exam is a routine examination that must be performed as part of the yearly physical examination, and testing the stool for blood is a routine part of this examination. In fact, the stool should be tested for blood twice a year. It is a very simple test and it could save lives.

RECOMMENDATIONS TO FOLLOW TO AVOID GETTING COLORECTAL CANCER

One should eat a diet that contains less saturated fat, and refrain from drinking liquids colored by any dye (red, yellow, green, pink). Also, one should eat a lot of fruits, stay away from seasoning food with a lot of artificial seasonings (as these may contain carcinogens or cancer promoters). Buy natural seasoning in the supermarket or make your own seasoning. Season food with natural lemon, lime or buy natural green or black pepper. Buy a lot of natural greens (as they do in the Tropics) to season food. Bear in mind that people who live in the Third World countries where they don't have access to fancy, expensive, modern seasoning and fat containing material, don't die of cancer of the colon and the rectum very frequently. Also, cancer of the colon is not very prevalent in the Third World countries because the people are poorer and don't eat rich, expensive foods. Stay away from too much red meat. Eat a lot of chicken (boil the chicken to remove the antibiotics and other material) and fish. If you can't afford expensive fish, just buy reasonably inexpensive fish. It is much better and healthier than red meat.

Recently, some reports came out suggesting that certain vitamins such as Vitamin C, Vitamin E and Vitamin A, when taken by mouth, may increase the membrane integrity of the lining of the esophagogastric junction, thereby reducing the incidence of cancer of that particular area, especially for those people who are alcoholics. It is documented that alcoholics and smokers have a high incidence of cancer of the esophagogastric junction. The cells in that area are damaged by the ir-

ritability that is caused by the effect of alcohol ingestion. It is believed that Vitamin C and Vitamin E, and possibly Vitamin A, can prevent the cellular abnormality that occurs as the result of the damage done to this area of the GI tract.

VITAMIN C AND ITS POTENTIAL ADVERSE EFFECTS ON GASTROINTESTINAL MALIGNANCY

There is a craze about taking vitamins which, by themselves, have a lot of problems. The truth is you don't need to take vast amounts of vitamins unless you have been documented to be vitamin deficient. Because, if you are not documented to be vitamin deficient and you are taking vitamins, you are just wasting your time and money because there is no place for the vitamins to go in the body.

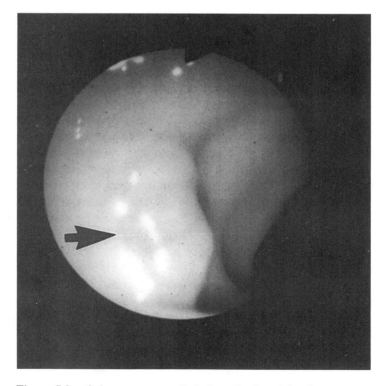

Figure 5.9. Colon cancer: sessile lesion of colon. (arrow)

The way vitamins work in the human system, you can only get value from the vitamins if the vitamin has a deficient place in the body for it to do the work that it is supposed to do. As long as you eat a good diet there is no reason for you to be taking all these unnecessary vitamins. Vitamins can hurt you more than they can help you. Later on I will mention where I think that vitamins have certain values, but, in terms of taking vitamins because you think they will make you strong, is false. It does not do it at all, regardless of what the vitamin industry says. There have been ample reports supported by the government and other scientific and academic institutions that document that. Taking large quantities of vitamins can, in fact, hurt you rather than help you. Even taking iron without it being documented by a physician that you are iron deficient, can be harmful. There is a disease called idiopathic hemochromatosis which is a hereditary condition whereby people over-absorb iron. If you take iron without being iron deficient, and if you happen to have this condition, you will over-absorb iron that will be stored in your heart muscle and your pancreas and in your liver. It could cause cirrhosis of the liver. It could damage the pancreas leading to secondary diabetes and it could give you an enlarged heart causing cardiomyopathy leading to early death, secondary to unexplained enlargement of the heart and heart failure. It is interesting to realize that Vitamin C will make this situation worse. Vitamin C is an important vitamin, it prevents scurvy and one has to ingest it because the body does not make it. Vitamin C, when taken in more than 500 mg., has the ability of causing you to over-absorb iron and also over mobilizing iron into the heart muscles

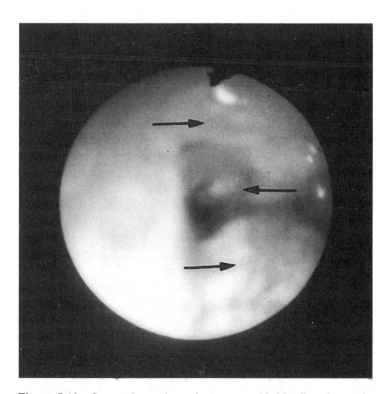

Figure 5.10. Large obstructing colon cancer with bleeding. (arrows)

and into the pancreas leading to damage to these organs that can lead to your death. So, taking Vitamin C can be extremely dangerous, unless you have been documented to be deficient in Vitamin C. In this country, it is very hard to find Vitamin C deficiency because the daily requirement for Vitamin C is only 60 mg. which can be reached by drinking a glass of orange juice. There are people who are taking as much as 1,000 mg. of Vitamin C per day because they are convinced that it helps them. In fact, they are throwing money away because there is no evidence that Vitamin C needs to be taken in that large a dose to deal with any known medical problems. Vitamin C does nothing for the common cold. The only instances in which one can justify taking Vitamin C are:

SOME POSITIVE EFFECTS OF VITAMIN C ON THE HUMAN BODY

1. If an elderly person has atrophic gastritis and is documented to be iron deficient, then Vitamin C can be added in a dose of 250 mg. three times per day to help reduce iron from ferric to ferrous to facilitate better absorption.

2. Vitamin C is said to be able to protect the tissues of the esophagogastric area, along with Vitamins A and E, from the development of cancer, especially in individuals who abuse alcohol and tobacco.

On the down side, taking Vitamin C can cause a false negative hemoccult test of the stool which can lead to the failure in the diagnosis of occult bleeding in conditions

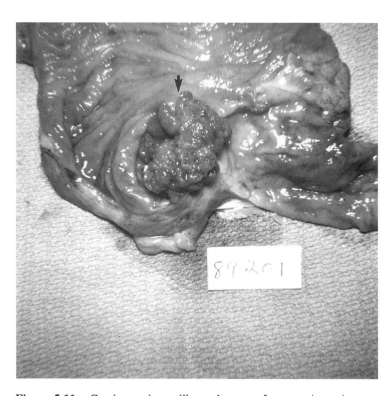

Figure 5.11. Carcinoma in papillary adenoma of cecum. (arrow)

such as ulcer of the stomach, stomach cancer and colorectal cancer. This occurs because Vitamin C is a reducing agent and the hemoccult test reaction is an oxidation reaction, so when Vitamin C is present, it neutralizes this reaction, causing it to be falsely negative. One must refrain from taking Vitamin C for 3 to 4 days before having his or her stool tested. Other substances that must be refrained from prior to having the hemoccult stool test done are aspirin and red meat. In the case of aspirin, one should stay off it from a week to ten days and for red meat, 3 to 4 days.

THE INCIDENCE OF LUNG CANCER

The total lung cancer statistics for 1991 (according to the American Cancer Society) is 161,000. Of this number, 101,000 men are expected to develop lung cancer in 1991, and 60,000 women are expected to develop lung cancer in 1991.

In 1991, 143,000 individuals are expected to die from lung cancer, 92,000 male and 51,000 female. In 1991, more women will die of lung cancer as compared to breast cancer. 51,000 women will die from lung cancer as compared to 44,500 women who are expected to die from breast cancer which means that 6,500 more women will die of lung cancer compared to breast cancer and, as mentioned before, in 1989, 21% of estimated cancer deaths in women was due to lung cancer and 18% was due to breast cancer. In 1989, 25% of men who died from cancer in the United States of America, had died from lung cancer.

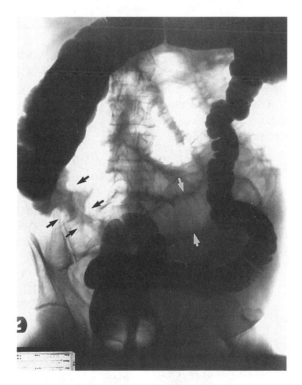

Figure 5.12. Barium enema: apple core lesion of the cecum (black arrow), with small bowel obstruction (white arrows).

When one compares the 5-year survival chance (published from 1979–1984 by the American Cancer Society, cancer statistics), one finds that in all stages of cancer of the lung there is a 13% 5-year survival chance in Whites, and only an 11% 5-year survival chance in Blacks. However, 33% of Whites presented with a localized lesion, but only 27% of Blacks presented with the same lesion of the lung.

THE DIFFERENT TYPES OF LUNG CANCER

There are several types of cancer. The most common types are: small cell cancers of the lung, known as oat cell carcinoma, adenocarcinoma, and squamous cell carcinoma. These are divided into two groups: small cell (oat cell) and large cell (a combination of all the large cell cancers).

Other types of cancers that can be found are cancers associated with exposure to asbestos, and cancer that develops as a result of working in the coal mines.

Of all things suspected to cause cancer, the one that has a definite proven association is cigarette smoking. Cigarettes not only cause cancer, but can cause emphysema, and coronary artery disease. Emphysema is a devastating disease because it causes a great deal of disability in the individuals who suffer from it. Heavy smoking is also associated with peptic ulcer disease because the nicotine in the cigarettes is a stimulant to acid production. Therefore, there is a high incidence of ulcers of the stomach in individuals who also have chronic bronchitis.

CIGARETTE SMOKING, ALCOHOL ABUSE AND CANCER OF THE OROPHARYNX

Cigarette smoking in association with alcohol abuse has a high incidence of cancer of the oropharynx, head and neck. Individuals who are involved in habits such as chewing and snuffing tobacco are succeptible to cancer of the pharynx because of the chemicals that are found in the tobacco.

THE HIGH INCIDENCE OF SMOKING IN BLACKS AND LUNG CANCER

It has been documented that the incidence of smoking in Blacks is higher than in the white population. Therefore, Blacks have a disproportionate incidence of cancer of the lung, secondary to heavy cigarette smoking. As it is for other types of cancer, Blacks almost always present to the doctor with this cancer in a more advanced stage, than their white counterparts. The reasons are either that they don't go to the doctor soon enough, or they ignore the symptoms (chronic cough, pain in the chest, shortness of breath). By this time they present themselves to be evaluated and have a chest x-ray, almost always the cancer is found in an unresectable stage.

LARGE CELL CARCINOMA OF THE LUNG

Large cell carcinoma of the lung, if found at the point where it is a coin lesion and can be resected. It is a curable disease. However, the same cannot be said about small cell carcinoma (oat cell) because it is a very peculiar disease. By the time it is discovered, no matter how small the lesion in the lung, it is almost always certain to already have distant metastases. The peculiarity of this tumor is why it is such a difficult disease to cure.

HOW TO APPROACH SOMEONE WITH AN ABNORMAL LESION IN THE LUNG AND CANCER IS SUSPECTED?

The first thing to do is a chest CT and then a complete physical examination. The patient should be bronchoscoped and biopsy taken to try to determine if the lesion in the lung is cancerous or not.

DIAGNOSING LUNG CANCER

Cancer of the lung can also be diagnosed by a cytology of the sputum. A fresh morning sputum is collected, and, by the cytology, one can determine if it is cancerous or not. However, the diagnosis cannot be made by only a bronchoscopy; one may choose to do a mediastinoscopy with biopsy. The lesion can also be approached by expert needle biopsy.

Once the biopsy is done, it can be determined whether or not the lesion is cancerous. The next step is to do an evaluation to look for metastases. To do this, a complete blood chemistries (to examine the liver functions), a bone scan, a CAT scan of the abdomen (to examine the liver to look for metastases), and a CAT scan of the brain (to examine brain metastases) is needed. If these are all negative, then the patient should be referred to an oncologist (who may have already been involved in the case) to arrange for treatment. If it is a large cell carcinoma, and it is a coin lesion, sometimes it can be resected. And, after the resection, a decision as to whether radiotherapy or chemotherapy should be provided has to be made. This decision usually depends on the stage and size of the tumor and should be made based on the particular case in question. If it is determined that it is a small cell carcinoma, once the evaluation is performed and metastases is found, the next step is combination chemotherapy.

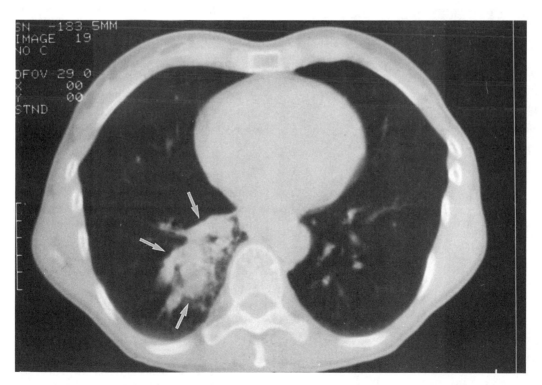

Figure 5.13. CAT SCAN of the chest lesion in inferior segment of left lower lobe of lung: squamous cell carcinoma (cancer) in a smoker. (arrows)

THE DIFFERENT TYPES OF CHEMOTHERAPY IN THE TREATMENT OF LUNG CANCER

Different types of combination chemotherapy are available. But, it depends on the individual setting where the patient is being treated. The type of approach to use to treat this particular type of patient with a particular type of chemotherapy depends on whether it is in the research setting or it is in the community hospital.

Several types of chemotherapy are available; for small cell carcinoma—a combination of Cytoxan, Adriamycin and VP 16 is one type of protocol. Or, a combination involving Cisplatin, VP16 is another type of protocol. There are other protocols that include Methotrexate and Procarbazine. Again,

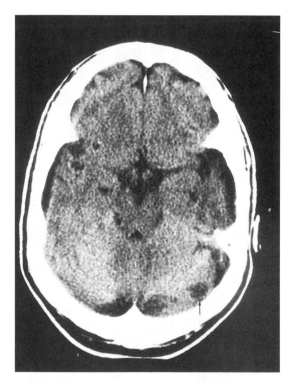

Figure 5.14. CAT SCAN of the Brain: Hypodense Mass Left Cerebellar hemisphere (arrow) Metastatic cancer to the brain from a lung primary in a smoker.

it depends on the oncologist and the individual case how to proceed to organize this combination of chemotherapy.

As for large cell carcinoma of the lung, combinations include: Cisplatin and VP 16 which work extremely well. Or, other combinations include: Velban with Cisplatin which also works rather well. Sometimes, radiotherapy is given first, and after an appropriate rest period (2–3 weeks to allow the marrow to recover) then, chemotherapy can be added. Also, large cell carcinoma of the lung is a potentially curable disease if diagnosed while it is a so-called coin lesion when it can be resected and surgically treated.

In summary, there is a higher incidence of cancer of the lung in Blacks and their white counterparts. Also, there is a higher incidence of smoking in the Blacks and other minorities. If one smokes, inevitably he/she is going to eventually develop cancer, heart disease or emphysema or a combination of any of the above.

CANCER OF THE OVARY

In 1991, according to the American Cancer Society statistics, 20,700 women are expected to develop cancer of the ovary, and of that number, 12,500 are expected to die of this cancer.

In 1989, cancer of the ovary represented 4% of the total number of cancers in the United States, and 5% of the total cancer deaths was due to cancer of the ovary.

When one compares the 5-year survival rate of white females as compared to Black females, in terms of all stages of ovarian cancer, the 5-year survival rate for white females is 37% and for Black females 36%. This is not much of a difference. However, 83% of the white females present with localized lesions as opposed to 79% of Black females, a significant difference. The reasons are once again the same, the Black females

86

always present with a lesion that is far more advanced than their white counterparts.

Cancer of the ovary is a very difficult cancer to diagnose because women complain of abdominal pains frequently, and almost always when they present with the cancer, it is significantly advanced. The recommendation is for frequent GYN examinations, palpation of the ovaries, and frequent pelvic sonograms associated with a pelvic examination. All of this is an attempt to discover if there is a mass in the ovary. If one is found, appropriate laparoscopy or other type of procedure should be performed so that the cancer can be detected and treated in its earliest stage. The chemotherapy available for cancer of the ovary today is much more encouraging than it has been in the past.

CHEMOTHERAPY IN OVARIAN CANCER

A combination of Adriamycin, Cytoxan and Cisplatin, added to examethylmelamine, has increased the overall cure rate in cancer of the ovary. Women, who suffer from cancer of the ovary, in the range of about 30–35%, are being cured by this combination chemotherapy. Twenty years ago, treatment for this cancer was dismal, but now if detected early, there is significant progress that has been made with combination chemotherapy.

CANCER OF THE CERVIX

Cancer of the cervix, if detected early, is also a treatable disease. However, if the cancer is detected at an advanced stage, it

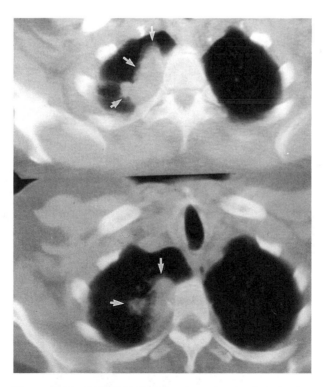

Figure 5.15. CAT SCAN of the chest showing lobulated mass (cancer) in the right upper lung in a patient who smokes (arrows)

becomes a very difficult cancer to treat and cure. The statistics published by the American Cancer Society in 1991, show that 13,000 women are expected to develop cancer of the cervix and 4,500 women are expected to die of this cancer. To diagnose cervical cancer is to perform a cervical pap smear. The pap smear is very accurate when performed appropriately. The pap smear is graded from Class I through Class IV. Class I is normal, whereas Class II would be somewhat abnormal (but this particular abnormality can sometimes be associated with inflammation, infection, etc.). If found, it is best that first the inflammation and infection be treated, and then the pap smear should be repeated to see if conditions have reverted to Class I. If conditions persist in being Class II, then the patient should be sent to the gynecologist for appropriate evaluation with biopsy.

DIFFERENT CLASSES OF PAP SMEAR

Also classes III (dysplasia), classes IV (carcinoma in situ) and classes V (invasive carcinoma) require biopsy. Carcinoma of the cervix has four different stages. Surgery or radiation therapy is considered effective treatment for stages I or IIA carcinoma of the cervix. Stages IIB, III and IVA are treated with radiation therapy. Whether or not hysterectomy is done in the treatment of the different stages of carcinoma of the cervix is left to the judgement of the individual physician. There is no effective chemo therapy in the treatment of cervical cancer.

RECOMMENDATIONS FOR PAP SMEAR

It is recommended that a woman has a pap smear once a year or, based on the re-

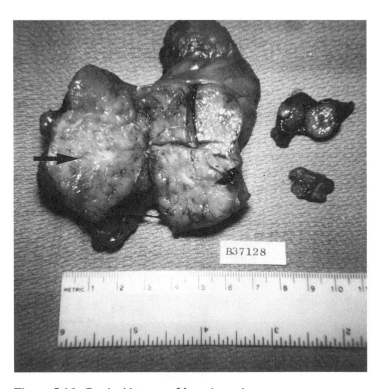

Figure 5.16. Carcinoid tumor of lung (arrow)

DIFFERENT CLINICAL STAGES OF CERVICAL CANCER

Preinvasive Carcinoma

Stage 0	Carcinoma in situ, intraepithelian carcinoma. Cases of stage 0 should not be included in any therapeutic statistics for invasive carcinoma

Invasive Carcinoma

Stage I	Carcinoma strictly confined to the cervix (extension to the corpus should be disregarded).
Stage Ia	Microinvasive carcinoma (early stromal invasion).
Stage Ib	All other cases of stage I. Occult cancer should be marked ''occ.''
Stage II	The carcinoma extends beyond the cervix, but has not extended on the pelvic wall. The carcinoma involves the vagina but not the lower third.
State IIa	No obvious parametrial involvement.
Stage IIb	Obvious parametrial involvement.
Stage III	The carcinoma has extended on the pelvic wall.
	On rectal examination there is no cancer-free space between the tumor and the pelvic wall.
	The tumor involves the lower third of the vagina.
	All cases with a hydronephrosis or nonfunctioning kidney should be included, unless they are known to be due to other cause.
Stage IIIa	No extension on the pelvic wall
Stage IIIb	Extension on the pelvic wall and hydronephrosis or nonfunctioning kidney.
Stage IV	The carcinoma has extended beyond the true pelvis or has clinically involved the mucosa of the bladder or rectum.
	A bullous edema as such does not permit a case to be allotted to stage IV.
Stage IVa	Spread of the growth to adjacent organs.
Stage IVb	Spread to distant organs.

Adopted in 1976 by the International Federation of Gynecology and Obstetrics

Source: Cancer—Principles & Practice of Oncology
      Volume I, 2nd Edition —Vincent T. Devita, Jr. et al

cent data, once every two years, but it is a crucial test for women to have performed to detect early cancer. Any woman who is sexually active ought to have a pap smear performed on a regular basis (once every 1 or 2 years). In the elderly, pap smears are also necessary as part of a complete physical examination. It is always important when performing a Pap smear to get a vaginal pool and a cervical smear. A vaginal pool is also necessary to rule out the possibility of cancer involving the vaginal wall itself. This is the reason why two smears are taken; one should be marked "C" for cervix, and the other identified as "V" for vagina.

As in a whole host of other cancers, the incidence of cervical cancer is mostly found in a more advanced stage in Black women as opposed to their white counterparts. In White women, it is 88% localized disease, and 84% localized disease in Black women. This is because Black women usually do not seek treatment until the cancer is far more advanced.

In all stages of cervical cancer, White females have a 67% 5-year survival rate; Black females, a 59% 5-year survival rate. Because Black women have Pap smears less frequently, cancer is usually detected in a far more advanced stage, thus the lower 5-year survival rate in all stages of cervical cancer.

CANCER OF THE ENDOMETRIUM

Furthermore, cancer of the endometrium, and of the uterus, again, is usually detected earlier in the white female, as compared to the Black female. In 1991, it is expected that 33,000 women in the United States will develop cancer of the endometrium and that 5,500 of these women are expected to die from this cancer.

DIAGNOSING CANCER OF THE ENDOMETRIUM

Cancer of the endometrium is diagnosed by a pelvic examination with appropriate Pap smears. If the woman is having symptoms of unexplained bleeding (bleeding in-between menses, which is abnormal), this should lead to the suspicion of cancer. D & C (dilation and curettage) should be performed with the appropriate scraping of the endometrium so the tissue is removed and evaluated microscopically and it shows evidence of cancer, then, it is confirmed that the patient has cancer of the uterus. Then, the appropriate surgical procedure, (a hysterectomy),

CLINICAL STAGING OF CARCINOMA OF THE ENDOMETRIUM

Stage 0		(TIS)	Carcinoma in situ
Stage I		(T1)	Carcinoma confined to the corpus
	IA	(T1a)	Uterine cavity 8 cm or less in length
	IB	(T1b)	Uterine cavity greater than 8 cm in length
			Stage I should be subgrouped by histology as follows:
			G1, highly differentiated, G2, moderately differentiated, G3 undifferentiated
Stage II		(T2)	Extension to cervix only
Stage III		(T3)	Extension outside the uterus but confined to true pelvis
Stage IV		(T4)	Extension beyond true pelvis or invading bladder or rectum

(Rubin P [ed]: Clinical Oncology for Medical Students, 5th ed, p 109. American Cancer Society, 1978)
Copied from Cancer, Principles & Practice of Oncology Second Edition, Vincent T. DeVita, Jr. et al

should be performed by a highly trained on-conological oncologist.

PRE-OPERATIVE EVALUATION FOR ENDOMETRIAL CANCER

Pre-operative evaluation consisting of abdominal CAT scan, barium enema and chest x-ray along with complete blood count and chemistries and coagulation profile i.e. PT and PTT should be done. Also, this specialist should prepare the patient for appropriate surgery with proper nodal dissection etc. to rule out the possibility of involvement of the node. This procedure can stage the disease to a point where postop radiation therapy vs. chemotherapy will be determined based on the stage that is found at surgery.

CLINICAL MANAGEMENT OF ENDOMETRIAL CANCER

Stage IA lesions are by and large treated with total abdominal hysterectomy with bi-lateral salpingo-oophorectomy with whole pelvis radiation added at the appropriate post-op period. All other stages of endometrial carcinoma are treated with a combination of surgery with radiation therapy. Combination chemo therapy consisting of Cisplatin, Adriamycin and Cyclophosphamide provide reasonably good response for patients endometrial cancer.

In cancer of the endometrium, (based on the latest published statistics by the American Cancer Society), the white female has an 83% 5-year survival rate in all stages of the disease at presentation while the Black

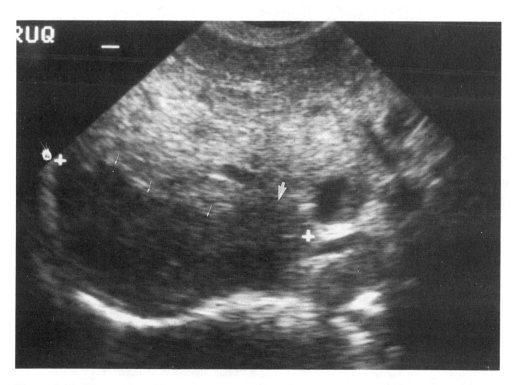

Figure 5.17. Ultra sound of liver showing metastatic cancer from a lung primary in a smoker (small and large arrows)

91

female has only a 53% 5-year survival chance. This is a 30% difference, which is a large percentage difference between the Black female as compared to the white female.

LOCALIZED CANCEROUS LESIONS IN BLACK VS. WHITE PATIENTS

If the patient has a localized lesion, the white female has a 91% 5-year survival rate as compared to 71% 5-year survival rate in the Black female. This is a 20% difference. The problem is Black females tend to present to their doctors less frequently to complain of the fact that she is having abnormal menstrual bleeding. And, she is less likely to go to a more specialized doctor because she cannot afford one. Also, she frequently goes to neighborhood clinics that are not very well equipped, and the health care practitioners are much less specialized to provide the appropriate care that is needed to diagnose the disease at an early stage. These are some of the reasons why there is a 30% difference between the 5-year survival rate of the white female (82%) as compared to the Black female (53%). Certainly, it shows the difference between the health care the Black female receives, as opposed to the white female. The white female is also more informed as to what may be wrong when she is having abnormal bleeding. She probably reads more appropriate journals where these types of abnormalities are described as opposed to the Black female who, if she has time to read, reads popular magazines that are less informative.

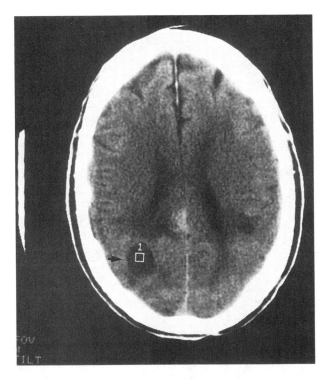

Figure 5.18. CAT SCAN of the brain showing metastatic cancer mass in para vantricular white matter from lung cancer in a smoker.

THERE IS NO GENETIC EXPLANATION AS TO WHY THE INCIDENCE OF CANCER IS HIGHER AMONG BLACKS THAN AMONG WHITES

Genetics have nothing to do with the predisposition to any particular carcinogen. The fact that women use different types of douching materials may play a role by causing some abnormality, but although these different solutions may cause infection by killing the bacteria (allowing the fungus that live in the vagina to grow disproportionately), are not cancer causing substances. Although anything that irritates on a continuous basis can cause dysplasia, (the dysplasia can go on to cause problems), there is no definite evidence that the douching agents themselves are cancer causing substances. It is important, however, to just use water to douche a day or two after a woman has a period to remove the excess blood. And, it is not necessary to use a corrosive agent. If a woman sees that she is having an abnormal discharge, she should not take it upon herself to use lysol and vinegar or other types of solution to douche. She should go to the gynecologist and let him/her evaluate the discharge through vaginal cultures and Pap smears, and then provide the appropriate treatment.

HIGHER INCIDENCE OF BREAST CANCER IN BLACK WOMEN

There is a higher incidence of breast cancer in African-Americans ages 40–45 in part due to the fact that black women tend to be more obese than their white counterparts. The role obesity plays is significant because the breast is being exposed to an overabundance of estrogen stimulation. Estrone, a precursor of estrogen, is found in adipose tissues (fat tissues) in the abdomen, thighs and buttocks and can be converted, under the influence of the adrenal glands, into estrogen. Estrogen, in turn, causes increased stimulation of the breasts which predisposes the breast tissues to the development of cancer. As a result, there is a higher incidence of cancer of the breast in obese women, especially Blacks who have a genetically transmitted gene that causes low basal metabolism. Low basal metabolism results in the inability of an individual to burn up ingested carbohydrates, which in turn leads to an increased carbohydrate store in the liver which then is converted into fat which settles in the muscles leading to obesity. Four hundred years ago or so, the fore-bearer of negroes in the new world allowed this low basal metabolism gene to develop in Black women of Africa. In an attempt to please their men, these women made every effort to be obese, and remain obese, because it is said that obesity in Africa, at that time, was a sign of beauty in women; so, the Black women's body adapted to that new obese body environment, passing down the gene to their offsprings, who, in turn, become obese, and so on and so forth. In other words, obese parents are expected to give birth to obese children, thereby perpetuating the obesity gene. Cervical cancer, endometrial cancer, both of these types of cancers are curable diseases if detected at an early stage. And, women need to be more vigilant in going to a doctor when they are having lower abdominal discomfort, unexplained vaginal discharge, and unexplained bleeding in-between periods. Also, if they are having prolonged bleeding during periods and unusual pain during intercourse. All these symptoms should prompt the woman to go to seek medical care for appropriate examination. These are: Pap smears, vaginal exams, pelvic sonograms, and appropriate D & C's to evaluate the tissue so that if cancer is present, it can be detected early. Also, a cure can be provided when the disease is in the very early stage.

CANCER OF THE PANCREAS

Another cancer that is very insidious and difficult to treat is cancer of the pancreas. It affects both men and women almost equally. In 1991, it is expected that 28,200 individuals will develop cancer of the pancreas and 25,200 of these individuals will die of this cancer; broken down into 12,000 men and 13,200 women.

What makes cancer of the pancreas such a vicious cancer is the fact that it is very difficult to detect. Often, the patient complains of vague abdominal pain, and unless one is very vigilant to do an abdominal sonogram or abdominal CAT scan, it is easy to miss the cancer. By the time it is discovered, it is almost always in an advanced stage. If by chance one has cancer of the head of the pancreas, this can quickly lead to obstruction of the biliary tree leading to obstructive jaundice which oftentimes can lead to an early diagnosis. Again, by the time the cancer is large enough to cause obstruction of the biliary system, it is almost always difficult to resect and cure surgically. If it is in the body of the pancreas, again it is difficult to detect because it does not cause jaundice very easily unless it has already metastasized to the liver. Of course, in the tail of the pancreas, it is also difficult to detect because it does not often cause early jaundice. It causes poor appetite, weight loss, and sometimes, in very rare instances, blood can be found in the stool of someone with cancer of the pancreas. Also, this is not a very easily resectable cancer. Most of the time, cancer of the pancreas is fatal. It does not respond very well to chemotherapy. The chemotherapy that is presently being used is 5 FU, Adriamycin and Mitomycin-C in combination. This particular combination is referred to as FAM.

CANCER OF THE PROSTATE AND ITS CLINICAL SPECTRUM

In 1991, it is expected that 122,000 men will develop cancer of the prostate and that 32,000 of these men are expected to die of this cancer. But, cancer of the prostate is a curable disease if detected early.

To detect this cancer early, a man has to have a prostate examination performed, and if the prostate feels abnormal to the physician, then an appropriate biopsy is needed to conclude the diagnosis. There are also other tests that can be used to determine if cancer of the prostate is present, such as: PAP (Prostatic Acid Phosphatase), PSA (Prostatic Specific Antigen).

However, it is also reasonably easy to detect cancer of the prostate. There is a new technique where certain characteristics of the prostate gland if cancerous, can be demonstrated by trans-rectal sonogram. A biopsy should be performed simultaneously and with the sonographic visualization, so one can diagnose prostate cancer. Again, if detected early, surgery can be performed to eradicate the cancer quickly. However, if it is detected late, it is a devastating disease which has a very high predilection to invading the bone which causes tremendous bone pain. Also, prostate cancer goes to the liver frequently, which causes liver metastases. But, if prostate cancer is detected, the urologist (who is the surgeon involved in doing surgery for prostate cancer) has to evaluate the patient and determine the appropriate metastatic workup which should include: a CAT scan of the abdomen, blood chemistries, CBC's, skeletal survey and chest x-ray, which is important because cancer of the prostate goes to the chest, and to the lungs readily. It should be decided at this stage on what type of surgery is needed. It may be limited surgery to the prostate, or it may involve a radical surgical procedure. In the process of treatment of prostate cancer when the disease is already advanced and has invaded the bone, it may be necessary to use special radiation therapy into the prostate to kill the cancer. Or, sometimes it may be necessary to do an orchiectomy as a means of preventing the progression of the cancer by removing the testes. The testes produce androgen, and androgen is the hormone that feeds the prostate cancer promoting growth. An orchiectomy can, in some cases, prevent the progression of the disease.

There are many other treatments that are available in the management of patients with prostate cancer. Amongst them are: DES (diethylistilbesterol), Leuprolide acetate (Lupron depot) and Eulexin. Both Leuprolide acetate and Eulexin work via different mechanisms to shut off the production of androgen thereby preventing the growth of prostate cancer. There is no effective chemotherapeutic agents for treating prostate cancer.

HIGHER INCIDENCE OF CANCER OF THE PROSTATE IN BLACK MALES

There appears to be a higher incidence of cancer of the prostate in Black males as compared to white males. It has not been determined why this is so. Also, prostate cancer in the Black male seems to be a more aggressive disease than in the white male. Smoking is said to have some association with it, and there is a higher incidence of smoking cigarettes in Black males than in white males.

Ingestion of a lot of red meat leads to ingestion of hormone producing fat. This predisposes the prostate to a higher incidence of this type of fat substances that can lead to the production of more hormones which stimulate the prostate.

In terms of the incidence of prostate cancer in white males vs. Black males, the 5-year survival rate in prostate cancer in all stages in white males is 72% as compared to 60% 5-year survival rate in the Black males. This is a 12% difference, which is a very

substantial difference. When the disease is presented localized there is an 85% 5-year survival rate in prostate cancer in the white males and 79% 5-year survival rate in the Black male. Again, the same observation is to be made that prostate cancer is a more devastating disease in Black males. And, more Black males die of the disease than white males. Again, more Blacks present with the disease in a more advanced stage than the white counterpart. This is based on the fact that Black males do not go for physical exams as often as white males, and they don't have as frequent rectal exams, and prostate evaluations. Therefore, the later the disease is detected, the more advanced the stage of the disease is at presentation, the more difficult it is to cure.

RECOMMENDATIONS TO HELP DECREASE THE INCIDENCE OF PROSTATE CANCER IN BLACK MALES

Black males ought to think more consistently about the need to have a rectal exam so that prostate palpation may be performed, and if necessary, a prostate sonogram. If there is a cancer focusing in the prostate gland, it can be detected earlier.

ACUTE PROSTATITIS, CHRONIC PROSTATITIS, AND BENIGN PROSTATIC HYPERTROPHY

Cancer, of course, is not the only disease that involves the prostate. There is acute prostatis and benign prostatic hypertrophy that lead to urinary obstruction which leads to urinary tract infections in a male. The prostate gland is located at the neck of the bladder and it's only function is to secrete fluid that mixes with the semen during ejaculation. Sooner or later, a man's prostate gland will be hypertrophied and this enlargement of the prostate gland is likely to lead to bladder neck obstruction. This results in urinary retention leading to the need for trans-urethral prostatectomy to remove the excess tissue from the gland to prevent urinary obstruction. Acute prostatitis occurs when bacteria invades the prostate gland which then becomes swollen and painful. There may be pain in the testicles, urinary frequency, fever or chills. This condition is treated with antibiotics such as CIPRO, BACTRIM, and most recently, FLOXIN. Sometimes, acute prostatitis can occur recurrently in the same individual, leading to chronic prostatitis, resulting in the need for treatment by a urologist.

CANCER OF THE TESTES

Testicular cancer is a reasonably common cancer that is found in a younger age group in the early 20's up to the mid 40's. In 1991, it is expected that 6,100 men will develop testicular cancer and 375 men are expected to die of this cancer in 1991. The way to evaluate for testicular cancer is to evaluate the testes during a physical exam. And, if an abnormal lump or mass is discovered, then the man is referred immediately to the urologist. An appropriate biopsy should be performed with the appropriate blood tests, x-rays, CAT scans etc. If the biopsy is proven to be positive for cancer, there is a cancer marker which is the Beta HCG. It is a blood test that can be elevated in testicular cancer. There is a very good combination chemotherapy for cancer of the testes: Cisplatin, Bleomycin and Velban. However, it is important to realize that testicular cancer is subdivided into seminomas, embryocarcinoma, teratoma (seen more in adults), choriocarcinoma. There is also teratoma with embryonal carcinoma type component to it and other types of tumors. It is a very complex disease. Surgery usually involves an orchiectomy and appropriate nodal dissections and radiotherapy. However, this particular tumor is a curable disease if found at a very

early stage. When a physician examines a young man, he or she should keep in mind the possibility of testicular cancer and perform an appropriate evaluation of the testes to make sure that there is no lump that can be palpated. If one is palpated, then the patient is referred immediately to the appropriate specialist (a urologist) who will perform the appropriate surgical procedure and then the medical oncologist or the radiation oncologist will provide the appropriate chemotherapy or radiotherapy for this particular type of tumor. Today, important progress has been made in curing young men with testicular type of cancer of different subcategories.

BLADDER CANCER

Bladder cancer is another very troublesome cancer that is difficult to treat because it is not always very responsive to chemotherapy. Although there is a chemotherapy regimen that is available for cancer of the bladder, the 5-year survival rate is not very good. In 1991, 50,200 individuals are expected to develop cancer of the bladder and 9,500 of these individuals are expected to die of this cancer.

Cancer of the bladder often presents with blood in the urine; (either gross hematuria or microscopic hematuria). Anytime a person presents with gross hematuria, a thorough evaluation of the urological tract should be performed including an IVP, ultrasound and cystoscopy, to evaluate the reason for the hematuria. Urine cytology is also very effective in determining whether there is a cancer cell present or not. Once the cystoscopic exam is performed, the bladder, ureters, and kidneys are evaluated to try to explain why the hematuria has occurred. Hematuria can be due to a whole host of things including infections, stones, and polyps.

Microscopic hematuria in Blacks can be the result of sickle cell trait or sickle cell disease. Both sickle cell trait and sickle cell disease at times cause microscopic hematuria. Sickle cell anemia itself has a propensity to cause bleeding from the kidney. Also, in the man, it can cause priapism which can present with bleeding. So, whenever microscopic hematuria or gross hematuria is found in Blacks, in addition to performing the above mentioned exams (the IVP, the sonogram and CAT scan and cystoscopy), hemoglobin electrophoresis should also be performed for the possibility for the sickling phenomenon being responsible for the hematuria.

CLINICAL APPROACHES IN THE MANAGEMENT OF BLADDER CANCER

If cancer is discovered, then the urologist has to stage the patient, and perform a CAT scan of the abdomen and pelvis to determine the possibility of lymphatic involvement. The type and extent of the surgery are the decisions of the urologist. The role of the oncologist in this cancer is based on how advanced the cancer is in terms of nodal involvement before chemotherapy can be entertained in this setting.

5-YEAR SURVIVAL RATE IN BLADDER CANCER IN BLACK MALES VS. WHITE MALES

In latest data published by the American Cancer Society, Whites show a 77% 5-year survival rate in all stages of bladder cancer while for Blacks, it is only 56%. This is a very significant difference. When the disease is presented in a localized stage, there is an 88% 5-year survival rate in Whites and an 80% 5-year survival rate in Blacks, a difference of eight percentage points. Blacks present with some type of hematuria (that has been ignored) or pain in the bladder area with discomfort, and dysuria. There have been recurrent symptoms that could be a urinary tract infection or pressure in the suprapubic area that has been ignored.

The reasons are the same as those previously cited: Blacks' lack of knowledge as to when and limited options as to where to seek treatment for blood in the urine. When they do go for care, it is often given by under-trained professionals in clinics that are inadequately equipped to provide appropriate medical care. The disease progresses and by the time it is detected, it is oftentimes in an advanced stage. Hence, this very large disparity of 77% 5-year survival rate in all stages of the bladder cancer in Whites vs. Blacks' 56%.

RECOMMENDATIONS TO HELP DECREASE THE INCIDENCE OF BLADDER CANCER

If one is having recurrent symptoms of pain during urination (hesitation), not being able to finish passing the urine, or there is blood in the urine, go to the doctor immediately to be examined. Have a urinalysis performed to make certain that there is blood, and a urine culture to determine that it is not an infection. If it is not an infection, proceed to have an IVP performed to examine particularly the bladder, the ureters, and kidneys, in order to explain why there is blood in the urine.

Also, blood in the urine can oftentimes be due to such things as stones in the kidneys (as mentioned above). The important thing is to be evaluated immediately so that if what is wrong is in the category of cancer, it can be detected early, and early treatment can be provided.

TREATMENT OF BLADDER CANCER

After the appropriate staging is carried out, a decision should be made by the urologist whether the patient needs a total cystectomy, partial cystectomy, or a combination with lymph node dissection. Sometimes, the installation of chemotherapy inside the bladder, depending on the stage, and in an advanced cancer, a combination chemotherapy is needed. The most effective combinations include: doxorubicin plus cyclophosphamide and vinblastine in combination with Methotrexate. Also, there are some combinations that include Cisplatin.

CANCER OF THE STOMACH AND ITS CLINICAL SPECTRUM

Cancer of the stomach is a curable disease if found at an early stage when hemigastrectomy can be performed with the appropriate post surgical management with chemotherapy. In 1991, 23,800 cases of cancer of the stomach are projected to occur, and 13,400 individuals are expected to die of cancer of the stomach in 1991.

Cancer of the stomach oftentimes presents with symptoms of ulcers. When the patient comes in, an upper GI series is performed. If an ulcer is found to have the characteristics of a cancerous lesion, then the patient is endoscoped immediately with biopsy. The biopsy is immediately sent to the pathologist for evaluation.

If someone comes in with symptoms of peptic ulcer disease, another approach is to have the patient undergo an endoscopic exam, and simultaneously, a biopsy should be performed. If the biopsy is cancerous, then appropriate measures are needed.

If an upper GI is performed, and one sees an ulcer, the patient should be treated with H2 blockers (Tagamet, Zantac, Axid or Pepsid) and after 2 months of treatment repeat the upper GI. If the ulcer has not healed, then have the patient endoscoped and perform a biopsy. An ulcer that has failed to heal after 2 months may be a cancerous ulcer.

If the biopsy is positive, then the patient should be referred to the surgeon for an appropriate surgical procedure to resect the part of the stomach that is cancerous. A node sampling should be performed at the time of surgery to determine the stage of the disease.

Prior to surgery, an abdominal CAT scan is needed to examine the liver and other nodes in the area. Also, a bone scan and a chest x-ray should be performed to stage the patient. Also, it is good practice to have a CEA level baseline performed so that during postop, the CEA can be used to monitor the progress of the patient.

TREATMENT OF STOMACH CANCER

If cancer is found, the nodes are negative, and the margins are clean, then surgery could be a curable procedure without radiotherapy or chemotherapy. On the other hand, if there is invasion of the muscularis with positive node involvement, then the patient will require chemotherapy postop. The chemotherapy available and most effective in cancer of the stomach is 5 Fluorouracil in conjunction with Mitomycin C.

5-YEAR SURVIVAL RATE IN STOMACH CANCER IN WHITES VS. BLACKS

In terms of the 5-year survival rate in Whites as it relates to stomach cancer, in all stages of the disease in 5-year survival rate is 16%. In this instance, the Blacks 5-year survival rate is 17%. One percentage more than Whites.

If the lesion is localized, the 5-year survival rate for Whites is 57%; for Blacks it is 54%. Gastric ulcers are more likely to be cancerous than duodenal ulcers.

RECOMMENDATIONS TO HELP DECREASE THE INCIDENCE OF STOMACH CANCER

If one is having symptoms of pain in the stomach, and feeling weak, that person should go to his/her physician. Oftentimes, cancer of the stomach can be painless and the first sign that the person is sick is that they are feeling weak (which means that they are bleeding). An evaluation of the stool for blood and performing a CBC which shows the characteristics of iron deficiency anemia, and a serum ferritin level that is very low are stages that lead a physician to perform an upper GI series. The physician can evaluate for the possibility of ulcers, or evaluate for another pathology to explain the anemia. Oftentimes, this is how cancer of the stomach is discovered. The key is to present to the doctor early. So, if cancer of the stomach exists, it can be resected at its earliest stage (stage 1), which enhances the chances of cure.

CANCER OF THE ESOPHAGUS

Cancer of the esophagus is another common cancer. It is also a very devastating disease because it does not respond well to chemotherapy. It is projected that there will be 10,900 cases of cancer of the esophagus in 1991, and that 9,800 individuals are expected to die of this cancer.

However, this is a disease that can be diagnosed easily. If someone is having trouble swallowing (the food is not going down readily and there is choking). One should go to a doctor immediately to be examined. One should have an upper GI series performed with an esophagram to examine if there is a lesion in the esophagus. An evaluation with endoscopic exam will detect the abnormality, and appropriate biopsy should be performed. But, this is not a cancer that responds very well to even surgical resection. It is a very devastating disease that is oftentimes associated with heavy cigarette smoking and heavy alcohol abuse.

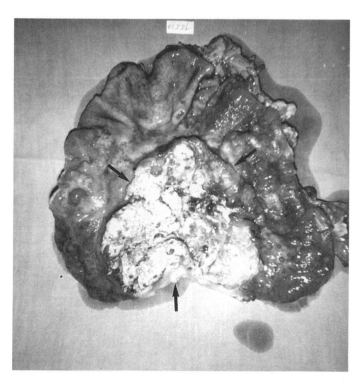

Figure 5.19. Gross pathology specimen from Cancer of the Stomach (arrows)

CANCER OF THE ESOPHAGUS AND ITS ASSOCIATION WITH CIGARETTE SMOKING AND ALCOHOL ABUSE

Individuals who smoke cigarettes and drink alcohol enhance their chances of cancer of the esophagus. Also, it is known that individuals who have had exposure to the ingestion of corrosive substances (lyes or acids) have a high incidence of cancer of the esophagus. The cure rate is very low, and the 5-year survival rate is very low, six percent in Caucasians, 5 percent in African-Americans. When the disease is localized it is 13% in Whites and only 8% survival rate in Blacks.

LYMPHOMA AND LEUKEMIAS

Also, there are a whole host of other malignancies that should be mentioned—such as Hodgkin's, Non-Hodgkin's lymphoma, leukemias (both non-lymphocytic and lymphocytic type). Leukemias have predilections for both the white and non-white population. Again, the trend is the same. Blacks and other minorities almost always present with this disease when they are in a more advanced stage than their white counterparts. Again, it is because of lack of education as to what to do when they become symptomatic. The key is that if one has nodes in the neck, or under the arm, or groin, that become very enlarged, and seem different, go and have these symptoms evaluated immediately so that appropriate biopsies can be performed with appropriate x-ray, to determine the cause for these types of malignancies.

If one is feeling very weak, this could oftentimes be the presentation of leukemias

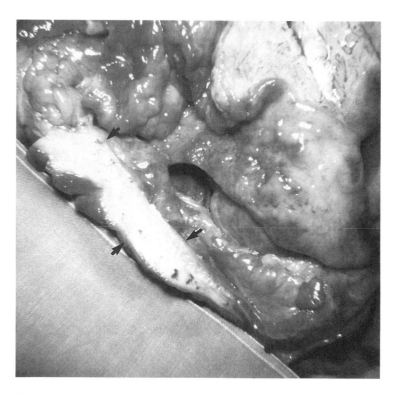

Figure 5.20. Gross pathology specimen from Cancer of the Stomach (arrows)

of different kinds. Also, fevers that are un-explained can be the presentation of leukemias or lymphomas. If one has these symptoms, go and have them evaluated. The projection is that in 1991 there will be 28,000 cases of leukemia and 18,100 individuals will die from this cancer. It is also projected that there will be 7,400 cases of hodgkin's disease and 1,600 individuals are expected to die of hodgkin's disease in 1991. It is also expected that there will be 37,200 cases of non-hodgkin's lymphoma and that 18,700 individuals will die of non-hodgkin's lymphoma in 1991.

SKIN CANCERS

Skin cancer in the United States is quite high; reported to be 600,000 cases per year. However, most of these cases of skin cancer are either basal cell or squamous cells. They are both highly curable with biopsies. The cancer of the skin that is the most serious is melanoma. It is expected that in 1991 there will be 32,000 cases of melanoma and 8,500 individuals are expected to die from this cancer. Melanoma is best treated with surgery if found early and radiotherapy also has a role to play. Chemotherapy has not been very effective and earlier claims made for immunotherapy have not stood the test of time.

MULTIPLE MYELOMA

Blacks have a high predilection of developing multiple myeloma and in Blacks, multiple myeloma is much more virulent. In 1991, it is expected that there will be 12,300 cases of myeloma and 9,100 individuals are

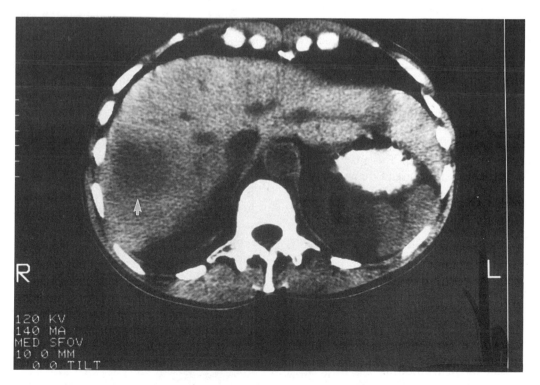

Figure 5.21. CAT SCAN of the abdomen showing metastatic lesion in the liver of a patient with cancer of the stomach (arrow)

expected to die from this cancer in 1991. Multiple myeloma causes anemia, renal failure, hypercalcemia, hyperviscosity and spontaneous bone fractures and a high rate of infections. Most people with myeloma die as a result of infectious and renal failure. The main stay in the treatment of multiple myeloma is prednisone, alkeran and radiotherapy when indicated.

CANCER OF THE BUCCAL CAVITY AND THROAT

Cancer of the buccal cavity and pharynx (lip, tongue, mouth and pharynx (throat) are much more common in Blacks than Whites because these cancers are associated with heavy smoking and heavy alcohol abuse and it is a known fact that Blacks smoke more than Whites and hence, the reason for the higher incidence of this type of cancer in Blacks. It is expected that in 1991 there will be 30,800 cases of buccal cavity and pharynx cancer and that 8,150 individuals are expected to die from this cancer in 1991.

SUMMARY

Cancer in 1991 is still a prominent disease. However, a large number of individuals, Whites and Non-Whites with different cancers, are being cured. The most important factor is early detection and treatment. Also, eat appropriate foods, stay away from foods and drinks that have coloring. Don't abuse alcohol, and refrain from cigarette smoking (which can cause lung cancer), stop eating foods that have too much grease, and stay away from too much red meat. Red meat is associated with the possibility of an increase in breast cancer in women and an increase in colon cancer in both men and women. Reorganize the diet. If there is not sufficient money to buy high grade food, try to intermix your foods with fruits and vegetables

(removing as much saturated fat as possible). One can basically lead a better and healthier life by decreasing the risk of developing cancer. As for women, at age forty have a baseline mammogram. At age fifty have a yearly mammogram. If there are cysts in the breasts, have the breasts examined 2–3 times a year. Thirty percent of women with breast cancer have had cysts, although there is no evidence that the cysts degenerate into cancerous lesions. But, cysts may cause confusion, and therefore a combination of breast exams and mammograms is needed to detect the possibility of cancer. If there is a family member with breast cancer, be more vigilant of the breasts by having more frequent exams.

If one smokes, have a chest x-ray (once a year or once every two years) and try to cut down, if not stopping completely, because smoking has a high association with cancer of the lung.

As for colon cancer and rectal cancer, don't ignore the symptoms. If one suddenly becomes constipated, or suddenly develops constipation alternating with diarrhea, and there is blood in the stool, then go to a doctor immediately to have an examination, a blood count, a serum ferritin, and undergo both sigmoidoscopic exam and a colonoscopic exam. When necessary, and when appropriate, x-ray exams such as barium enema are needed to determine whether or not there is a cancer of the rectum or colon. If one feels weak, go to the doctor to be evaluated so that this disease can be detected and appropriate care can be given early. This ensures the possibility of cure.

Again, the most important thing is early detection. If one is dissatisfied with the care one is receiving, make the effort to seek competent medical attention to eradicate the disease and possibly prolong one's life.

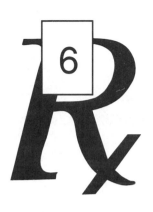

ALCOHOLISM AND ITS ASSOCIATED PROBLEMS IN AFRICAN-AMERICANS

CHAPTER OUTLINE

ALCOHOLISM AND ITS PROBLEMS

There are approximately 22 million alcoholics in the United States according to the National Council on Alcoholism. The projected monetary cost to the American society for problems relating to alcohol abuse in 1990 was approximately 36 billion dollars. This cost includes: medical problems, psychiatric problems, related crimes, accidents, and the loss of work. The problem of alcoholism affects the Black community and other minorities more severely than it affects the white population.

Blacks seem to start drinking at an early age, along with other minorities, now seem to have a chronic problem with alcohol abuse and all its associated social and economic devastation.

Alcohol is still the predominant drug abused in the American society. One reason for this is because it is so readily available, and one does not have to resort to illicit means to obtain it.

On a yearly basis, alcohol and its associated problems lead to approximately 100,000 deaths or more. Of this number, close to 40,000 are due to cirrhosis of the liver and the rest are due to accidental deaths, and homicides.

WHAT IS ALCOHOLISM?

Alcoholism is a disease and ought to be treated as such. It is a serious disease causing both psychological and medical complications. The psychological dependence on alcohol is real. It is well known that individuals who have alcohol problems are unable to stop drinking once they have started. They develop a psychological dependence on it. Individuals whose mothers and fathers were alcoholics have a higher likelihood themselves of becoming alcoholics. It is not quite clear as to whether this is due to a real genetic problem or just to the fact that they grew up in this environment. Because they were exposed to alcohol abuse, and they saw their parent drinking, they are more likely to drink to relieve stress, agitation, etc.

ALCOHOL ABUSE AND PEER PRESSURE

The issue of real peer pressure is why teen-agers are abusing alcohol. As there is peer pressure to get involved in illicit drugs, there is also peer pressure to force other young teen-agers to drink alcohol. For that matter, there is peer pressure in adults as well, to get together in a bar and drink. It seems that most alcoholics are not aware of the fact that they are alcoholics. But, if one drinks on a regular basis, then one eventually becomes dependent on alcohol.

UNDER THE INFLUENCE OF ALCOHOL

Being under the influence of alcohol is determined by the blood alcohol levels. Driving while impaired is when one has a blood level of 20 mg. per ml. At a blood level of 30 mg. per ml, one feels slightly disoriented. At a level of 50 mg per ml., there can be incoordination, (inability to walk a straight line), and at a level of 100 mg. per ml, one may have a more pronounced inability to walk, (actual stumbling). At a blood alcohol level of 100 mg. per ml., one would be driving while drunk, and at a blood alcohol level of 200 mg. per ml., one becomes confused, disoriented, and may even begin to lose consciousness, (blackout). A blood alcohol level of 400 mg. per ml. can actually result in coma and death.

ALCOHOL ABUSE

The amount of alcohol that it takes on a daily basis to cause damage to the liver is 80 grams of alcohol. Eighty grams of alcohol can be found in a 6-pack of 12 oz. cans of beer because each 12 oz. of beer has 13.1

grams of alcohol. If one multiplies this by 6 this results in 78.6 grams of alcohol which is pretty close to 80 grams per day. So, if one drinks this amount on a regular basis, the individual will develop liver disease as time goes on. If one drinks wine regularly, (3.5 fl. oz. glass of wine has 9.6 grams of alcohol) a bottle of wine usually has in the neighborhood of 5–6 glasses of wine. Hence, the reason why individuals who drink wine with their dinner, 2–3 glasses of wine per night, do not develop liver disease because it takes a minimum of 80 grams of alcohol for someone to begin to develop fatty infiltration which leads to metamorphosis of fat, leading to necrosis, leading to alcoholic liver disease with cirrhosis.

The same thing applies to champagne. One glass of champagne has 11 grams of alcohol in it, and some champagne has 13 grams depending if it's dry champagne. So, it really takes a tremendous amount of champagne on a daily basis to add up to 80 grams per day to give one liver disease from alcohol. However, if one drinks Martinis, this is a different situation. Each Martini has 18.5 grams of alcohol. So, if one drinks 5 Martinis per day, one is already drinking what is, in fact, in excess of the minimum amount that is needed to cause liver disease. A Manhattan, for instance, has 19.9 grams of alcohol which is a high concentration of alcohol. A Gin Ricky has 21.0 grams of alcohol. A Highball has 24 grams of alcohol which is very dangerous. A Mint Julep has 29.2 grams of alcohol. So, it does not take very many of these alcoholic drinks, on a daily basis, for someone to develop liver disease.

The important thing is to try to abstain from alcohol abuse altogether. If one drinks socially, try to limit the amount of alcohol consumed to less than 80 grams per day, so that liver disease does not develop. However, one has to understand that every organ in the human anatomy is sensitive to the direct effect of alcohol. And, some of these organs are affected by the secondary effects of alcohol. So, alcohol abuse is an addiction, and it leads to destruction of the vital organs.

Alcohol is destructive to the brain causing dementia. If the brain is mature, there may be an inability to function in one's occupation, or serious psychosocial problems along with other cognitive impairments such as significant memory loss. If all this affects an adult, then imagine what alcohol does to the unborn infant whose brain is just in the process of forming. It is extremely toxic to the brain tissue. It is known to cause the Korsakoff's syndrome (which is the result of vitamin deficiencies). It is also known to be associated with acute episodes of encephalopathy as a result of Wernicke's encephalopathy. It is also associated with all sorts of signs of abnormal neurological functions such as ataxia, (inability to walk a straight line) and other abnormalities such as eye movement abnormalities. Also, mood fluctuation with suicidal ideation can occur as a result of alcohol abuse and intoxication.

Another issue is that the person is not dangerous just to himself or herself, but is very dangerous to others in terms of driving while intoxicated. Or, being dangerous by attacking other individuals while under the influence which may result in trauma to self and to others. Also, a whole behavior change occurs in alcoholics.

ALCOHOL AND NUTRITION

What relationship does drinking alcohol have with nutrition? Does good nutrition prevent alcohol damage to the liver? The answer is no, because alcohol is directly toxic to the liver. If one is poorly nourished, naturally the overall situation of that person's anatomy is worse. The person will become weaker and become sick or infected faster. But, it does not matter how well one eats. If one consumes alcohol in excess, one is going to get sick from that amount of alcohol, because the alcohol is directly toxic to the liver.

Studies have been conducted where good nutrition vs poor nutrition was tried in baboons, who were given the same amount of alcohol. Both groups of animals wound up having the same degree of liver damage. It really does not matter if one eats well or one eats poorly. Naturally, if one eats poorly, the overall condition will become worse. One is likely to become sicker quicker. But, regardless of how well one eats, one is going to become sick if one abuses alcohol.

BLOOD TESTS IN ALCOHOL ABUSE

In addition to measuring the blood level, to determine if somebody has been drinking, the most sensitive test for this is the Gamma Glutamyl TransPeptidase (GGTP). If one were to have 6 cans of beer or 4–5 drinks the night before, the GGTP would be elevated the next morning because it reflects fatty liver and other infiltrative processes of the liver.

Mean Corpuscular Volume

Another test that is reasonably sensitive to determine whether someone has been drinking is the mean corpuscular volume (MCV). The normal is 80–94 fl./L. However, anyone who drinks excessively has a folate deficiency. Because the alcohol is a direct poison to the body, it causes an effect to the folate pathway that leads to an increase of the MCV. These two factors can be detected immediately in an office setting if the doctor needs to know about a patient's drinking. Also, these two tests can be a verifiable indication of the extent of alcohol that has been consumed.

MEDICAL PROBLEMS ASSOCIATED WITH ALCOHOLISM

In addition to the serious problems involved with alcohol in terms of family trage-dies, homicides and violence, are the medical problems.

BLUNT TRAUMAS TO THE HEAD IN ALCOHOLICS

Alcohol abuse affects the brain by damaging the brain cells. In addition to damaging the brain cells which leads to organic brain syndrome, the effect of frequent drunkenness may lead to blunt traumas to the head. This leads to subdural hematomas, epidural hematomas, or skull fracture. These problems affecting the brain can lead to a focus in the brain that can be associated with seizures.

PERIPHERAL NEUROPATHY IN ALCOHOLICS

Another neurological problem associated with alcohol is peripheral neuropathy, which is damage to the peripheral nerves.

GASTROINTESTINAL TRACT PROBLEMS IN ALCOHOLICS

Another problem associated with alcohol and the gastrointestinal (GI) tract is gastritis. Alcohol-induced gastritis leading to severe gastrointestinal bleeding is a major problem in alcohol abuse. And, it can lead to massive GI bleeding that often times necessitates blood transfusions and other complications.

Mallory-Weiss Tear

Also, another major problem in the GI tract associated with alcoholism is the Mallory-Weiss tear. This is a tear that occurs in the esophagogastric junction as a result of retching, secondary to alcohol abuse, and vomiting. One can actually cause a tear that leads to severe bleeding which would necessitate emergency surgery. In some cases, one has to have a plication performed to stop the bleeding. Also, this may present a serious situation because it is usually attended to in an emergency setting on someone who is already in a poor medical condition.

Variceal Bleeding

Another problem associated with alcohol and upper GI bleeding is variceal bleeding. A varix is a neovascularization. This is a vessel that is involved with the surface of the upper GI tract and the esophagus. Because the regular vessels are blocked (due to cirrhosis of the liver and portal hypertension, the vessels within the liver are destroyed), a new vessel is formed superficially on the surface of the esophagus and upper stomach. These new vessels bleed very easily, and when they do bleed, they bleed profusely. It is very difficult to provide treatment for this condition because even surgery does not seem to help. Laser treatment has been tried and in some settings the use of Inderal has been prescribed. However, this type of bleeding on a recurrent basis eventually leads to death. When one puts a tremendous amount of blood in the GI tract and if the liver is functioning poorly, the individual eventually develops liver failure. This leads to hepatic encephalopathy which often times causes death.

Ulcers of the Stomach

Ulcers of the stomach are associated with alcohol abuse because alcohol is a gastric retardant. Alcohol may increase one's appetite when one drinks moderately. However, when one drinks alcohol in large amounts and then eats, it causes retardation of the digestive process. When the food in the stomach is not digested, greater amounts of acid is produced in an attempt to digest of food. The more acid that is needed, the more likely it is that one will develop hyperacidity, which leads to ulcers of the stomach.

In addition, these individuals may smoke. It is known that smoking is associated with a high incidence of ulcers of the stomach. So, smoking and drinking in combination may cause ulcers of the stomach, leading to severe bleeding.

LIVER DISEASE IN ALCOHOLICS

Alcohol is a direct toxin to the liver. It causes liver tissue damage, which leads to cirrhosis. Once cirrhosis occurs, the liver becomes partially destroyed. Liver damage leads to portal hypertension. And, portal hypertension results in neovascularization which may result in esophageal varices and also an enlarged spleen.

Hypersplenism

The enlarged spleen leads to what is called hypersplenism. Once one has an enlarged spleen with hypersplenism, there develops a situation whereby the spleen is taking away platelets, (white cells, and red cells) resulting in chronic hemolysis. Hypersplenism and pancytopenia are the result of chronic alcoholic liver disease, and this is a combination that may develop into a serious condition.

Once one develops a low platelet count, they may bleed readily due to minor traumas. Platelets are particles that are needed in the human body to seal a cut. If one's platelet count is low, there will not be sufficient platelets to seal a cut, resulting in continuous bleeding.

If one has a platelet count of 20,000 or below, one could bleed spontaneously whether there is a cut or not. With a platelet count anywhere from 50,000 to 60,000, and one is cut, it is likely that one will not stop bleeding because the platelets are too low. If someone develops gastritis, secondary to alcohol ingestion, and then develops bleeding on the surface of the stomach, because of a low platelet count, the bleeding may not be stopped. In these individuals, even if the platelets are replaced, the spleen is going to immediately absorb the platelets. Also, most coagulation factors are produced in the liver. If the liver is damaged, the liver cannot produce enough coagulation factors.

Therefore, these individuals will present themselves with an elevated prothrombin time, an elevated partial thromboplastin time and if they start bleeding, it won't stop because of coagulopathy, (abnormal coagulation). Also, they may have a thrombopathy, which is low platelets, which develops into continuous bleeding.

In addition to the abnormal coagulation, because of hypersplenism, alcohol can acutely lower the platelet count whether one does or does not have cirrhosis or an enlarged spleen. Consuming too much alcohol can cause acute alcoholic injury, i.e., thrombocytopenia, which also leads to significant bleeding. Also, alcohol is toxic to the white and red cells, and to the platelets. It can also acutely deplete bone marrow production, and, if one drinks a large amount of alcohol frequently, they may eventually develop acute pancytopenia associated with toxicity from the alcohol. This condition may not be associated with chronic liver disease, but it could cause the same results leading to the nonproduction of essential bone marrow. As a matter of fact, if one does a bone marrow test on someone who is acutely intoxicated, one is likely to see actual vacuoles (holes) in the immature red cell, mature megacaryocytes.

ALCOHOL ABUSE AND ITS EFFECTS ON THE PANCREAS

The pancreas is an organ that is needed to secrete insulin. Insulin is needed to metabolize sugar and other carbohydrates. The pancreas is also important because it secretes many other substances that are needed for proper digestion. When one eats anything that contains fat without a healthy pancreas, this substance will become like caster oil. It may cause constant diarrhea because of the inability to emulsify fat. The fat is not broken down because there is not enough proper substance secreted by the pancreas to digest the fat properly.

Acute Pancreatitis Due to Alcohol Abuse

The pancreas is an organ that is very easily and almost always damaged by individuals who drink alcohol excessively. Excessive alcohol leads to acute pancreatitis, which can lead to pseudocysts of the pancreas which can develop into other disastrous conditions. This can lead to chronic pancreatitis.

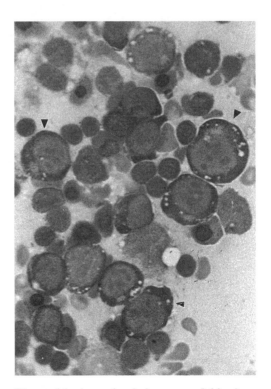

Figure 6.1. Arrow head shows megaloblastic red cells (large immature red cells) in a bone marrow of an alcoholic patient. The white dots within the large cells are vacuoles that are the result of alcohol toxicity. This picture is that of a folic acid deficiency as seen in an alcoholic resulting in macrocytic anemia.

At the point of chronic pancreatitis, the pancreas is no longer functioning sufficiently. It is scarred and damaged and causes frequent recurrent and persistent diarrhea because of malabsorption. One cannot absorb the food that is eaten because it is not digested.

Chronic Pancreatitis Due to Alcohol Abuse

This is the result of not having the proper enzymes to enable digestion. Not only does this condition cause frequent diarrhea, but one can also become secondary diabetic because of this damage to the pancreas. This is a form of diabetes mellitus that occurs secondary (due to the damage to the pancreas) because of alcohol abuse. So, alcoholism can cause havoc to the human body through many mechanisms and conditions. Also, individuals who drink and smoke cigarettes have a high incidence of cancer of the pancreas which is an incurable cancer 99% of the time.

DIFFERENCE IN THE EFFECTS OF ALCOHOL ABUSE IN DIFFERENT INDIVIDUALS

Different individual's bodies react differently to the toxic effect of alcohol. However, drinking in excess of 80 grams of alcohol per day, for about 7 years, is said to be sufficient to cause enough damage to the liver to lead to cirrhosis. In addition, it is also said that drinking in excess of 80 grams

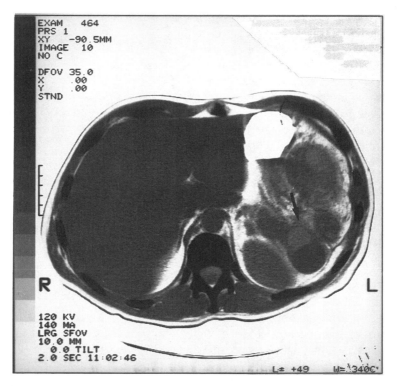

Figure 6.2. CT if the abdomin showing acute pancreatitis with a pseudocyst of the pancreas. (arrow showing swollen pancreas with pseudocyst)

of alcohol per day, for 7 years, will cause most individuals to develop acute pancreatitis. If one drinks the same amount of alcohol for a total of 14 years, then one is likely to develop chronic pancreatitis, and if one drinks the same amount of alcohol for another 7 years, totaling 21 years, then that usually adds up to the death of that individual. This is the so-called *law of seven* as it relates to chronic alcoholism. Needless to say, there are exceptions to this rule.

ALCOHOLISM AND ITS EFFECTS ON THE HEART

Alcohol abuse can cause severe diseases of the heart. There is alcohol induced cardiomyopathy because the muscle and the myocardial fibers become destroyed. Also,

alcohol abuse can cause an enlarged heart, which can result in congestive heart failure, and cardiac arrhythmias.

ALCOHOLISM AND ITS EFFECTS ON THE LUNGS

Alcohol can lead to diseases of the lungs because intoxication can cause the loss of the gag reflex, therefore, one aspirates very easily. This may develop into recurrent aspiration pneumonia which, if not treated properly, is deadly. In addition to this, alcohol causes immunosuppression. This means that frequent alcohol drinking causes the white cells to not function properly. Therefore, an individual who is an alcoholic is not really able to fight infection appropriately because he/she is indeed immunosuppressed.

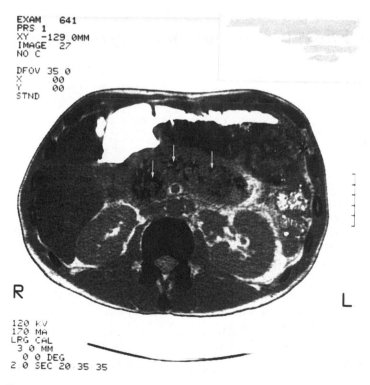

Figure 6.3. Cat Scan of the abdomen showing chronic pancreatitis with calcifications. Arrows showing swollen pancreas in a patient who abuses alcohol.

The white cells cannot migrate towards the site of infection properly. In addition, to developing hypersplenism which causes leukopenia and neutropenia, alcoholics are likely to have a lower white cell count that is not functioning properly, which leads to infection.

ALCOHOLISM AND HYPERTENSION

Alcoholism is associated with hypertension because when one is drunk (and is drunk repeatedly several times a week or almost every day), this results in a constant state of agitation. This constant state of agitation leads to hypersecretion of the catecholamines (epinephrine and norepinephrine). The sympathetic system becomes hyperactive causing a constant elevation of blood pressure. When blood pressure is high and if it is not brought down, it is going to affect the heart. The heart has to work that much harder to pump the blood forward. Therefore, alcoholic associated hypertension is another way to develop cardiovascular disease leading to atherosclerotic heart disease. Alcohol also contains carbohydrates which are associated with increased triglycerides which often results in coronary artery disease secondary to increased levels of triglycerides.

Blacks already have a high predisposition to essential hypertension leading to a high risk of strokes and cardiac disease secondary to coronary artery disease. Alcohol becomes another risk factor because it modulates the previous effect of untreated hypertension. It makes the hypertension worse. Hypertension is known to be associated with atherosclerotic disease of the vessels around the heart. When this is combined with a high level of triglycerides (a known risk factor for plaque formation), one clearly has a formula that can result in early death.

ALCOHOLISM AND ITS EFFECTS ON THE ENDOCRINE SYSTEM

Statistics show that more black women suffer from the effects of alcohol abuse and related health problems than African-American men. In the case of women, hormones are needed for proper functioning of the reproductive organs. One problem that may develop is with menstruation. When a woman is menstruating and is abusing alcohol, she can develop liver disease. She can have breakthrough bleeding causing excessive menstrual bleeding. The reason for this is that estrogen needs to be broken down by the liver. This doesn't occur if the liver is damaged. Therefore, if the liver is damaged and a higher level of estrogen is circulating in a woman's blood, this will cause excessive bleeding. In addition, because she has a high level of estrogen circulating in her blood, this predisposes her to develop breast cancer. The more frequently breast tissue is stimulated by estrogen, the more likely it is to become cancerous. And, similarly, the more the endometrium is stimulated by estrogen, the more the endometrium is likely to become cancerous. Therefore, a high estrogen level is not only associated with breakthrough bleeding, but it also leads to a high incidence of cancer of the uterus, and cancer of the breast. This is one endocrine problem that can be identified immediately related to alcohol abuse. Also, the inability to dispose of the estrogen leads to secondary changes in the sex characteristics of women who are abusing alcohol.

As for the men, they also develop problems because their livers are damaged. They are not able to break down the small amount of estrogen that their adrenals produce causing shrinkage in the glans penis, shiny small testicles, and gynecomastia (enlarged breasts). Again, all of this is due to the fact that there is too much estrogen circulating in the body, and the liver (because of alcohol related damage) is not able to break it down.

Secondary Hyperaldosteronism

Both men and women who drink excessively, develop secondary hyperaldosteronism. Secondary hyperaldosteronism causes the retention of too much salt. Also, those who have cirrhosis of the liver develop ascites, (a big abdomen with fluid), because of the liver's inability to break down aldosterone. Therefore, secondary hyperaldosteronism with high salt retention leads to fluid retention in the abdomen, and legs.

Alkalosis

If one develops alkalosis, he/she is also likely to have hypokalemia (low potassium) and high bicarbonate associated with it. This results in electrolyte abnormalities which can lead to cardiac arrhythmias and other aberrations leading to immediate death because of low potassium.

LIVER FAILURE AND INFECTIONS IN ALCOHOLICS

Liver problems associated with alcohol abuse are severe. Most of the individuals who are chronic alcoholics do not bleed to death but die as a result of liver failure. Also, they die of pneumonia secondary to infection because of aspiration, and the inability to fight infection. The infection is often brought on by hypersplenism, (a large spleen or the malfunction of the spleen). If the spleen is not functioning properly, one becomes more prone to be infected by a capsular organism, such as pneumococcus or H. flu. Alcoholics in particular have a tendency to be infected with Klebsiella pneumoniae. This is an organism that causes pneumonia because of aspiration, which occurs during episodes when they aspirate and vomit. This creates problems because of the inability to control the swallowing mechanism.

HEMATOLOGICAL PROBLEMS IN ALCOHOLICS

Also, hematological problems associated with alcohol abuse are severe. When someone has severe liver disease, one can develop anemia because of acute blood loss, secondary to acute bleeding. They can develop anemia secondary to chronic variceal bleeding leading to iron deficiency anemia, and they can develop anemia secondary to peptic ulcer disease which also leads to iron deficiency anemia. Also, alcoholism is associated with folate deficiency.

Folic Acid Deficiency

Folic acid deficiency is a serious form of anemia. It is serious because the patient who abuses alcohol may neglect to eat foods such as legumes which contain folic acid. The daily requirement for folic acid is 50 micrograms. Folic acid has to be taken on a regular basis in order for someone to remain in a folate balance. The body does not have the capability of producing folic acid on its own, therefore an individual must ingest folic acid. The anemia that folic acid causes is megaloblastic in characteristic.

B–12 VITAMIN DEFICIENCIES IN ALCOHOLICS

Vitamin deficiency also occurs in chronic alcoholics because of malabsorption. Recurrent malabsorption secondary to chronic pancreatitis can lead to B–12 deficiency. Also, alcoholics frequently develop peptic ulcer disease. The possibility of having to be operated on and removing a significant portion of the stomach exists, and this type of surgery often results in B–12 deficiency seven to ten years later.

People who drink chronically and heavily are deficient in all of the B vitamins. Therefore, these individuals have a lot of other associated signs of alcohol abuse, a big red tongue, and paresthesias (pins and needles in the muscles), as a result of nerve damage and a lack of sufficient B vitamins. They also suffer from a disease called pellagra, that is associated with lack of the B vitamins. The reason that they develop pellagra is because they are lacking Niacin. Also, pellagra can be associated with dermatitis and dementia, and diarrhea. Also, they can develop thiamine deficiency, which may lead to a disease called beri-beri. Chronic thiamine deficiency, (beri-beri) can also be associated with heart disease leading to high output failure.

Thiamine deficiency can cause serious nervous system abnormalities such as Wernicke's syndrome. This is a condition that is associated with the loss of sensation and the loss of motor reflex function.

Another vitamin deficiency that can occur is Vitamin B–6 which is pyridoxine. This occurs reasonably frequently in individuals who are severe alcoholics. Some of the signs of vitamin B–6 or pyridoxine deficiency, include glossitis, and as mentioned, a big red tongue, also, seborrheic dermatitis, and cheilosis (a slit on the side of the mouth).

Cheilosis can also be caused by iron deficiency but certainly B–6 deficiency is one of the major causes. Also, weakness and dizziness are associated with B–6 deficiency. Along with the other type of vitamin B deficiencies, there is a riboflavin deficiency which again can cause dermatitis and glossitis. However, do not take riboflavin as a vitamin by itself because it is extremely dangerous and an overdose can lead to death. When one is deficient from riboflavin, they may develop cheilosis, angular stomatitis, glossitis, and seborrheic dermatitis. Also, there is a normo-chromic normocytic type of anemia that is also associated with riboflavin deficiency. When one has vitamin B complex deficiency, they become deficient in riboflavin, vitamin B–6, thiamine, and Niacin.

MAGNESIUM DEFICIENCY IN ALCOHOLICS

Another deficient substance is magnesium. The lack of magnesium causes a calcium deficiency which can lead to seizures. Magnesium is needed in order for the parathyroid gland to work properly in the production of calcium. When one has magnesium deficiency (seen in most chronic alcoholics), they often times present with hypocalcemia which again can lead to seizures, because of the low calcium as a result of the low magnesium. Also, they lack phosphate.

PHOSPHATE DEFICIENCY IN ALCOHOLICS

Low phosphate can not only cause seizures but it could also cause hemolytic anemia. Low phosphate in the neighborhood of 1 to 1.5 can cause acute hemolysis of the red cells, known as hemolytic anemia.

HYPOGLYCEMIA IN ALCOHOLICS

Hypoglycemia is caused by the lack of sufficient food and blood sugar. It is a known fact that the diet of the minorities, in particular, poor blacks and Hispanics is very marginal. When they present to the Emergency Room, they frequently are in a nutrient and vitamin starved condition.

EMERGENCY ROOM SETTING AND THE TREATMENT OF ALCOHOLICS

When an alcoholic patient presents himself/herself in an Emergency Room setting, the first thing one does is to examine the patient immediately and thoroughly. Draw blood and send it for alcohol and drug screening. Before starting an IV, take a stat blood sugar, electrolytes, blood chemistries and a complete blood count. Once the drug screening has been processed and while one is waiting for the results of the CBC and chemistries, especially the blood sugar, start an IV. Start the IV with normal saline at first and then give the patient 100 mg. of thiamine. Then, give the patient 1 gram of magnesium sulfate and proceed to give the patient 50 cc's of 50% dextrose IV. This is because the patient is likely to be hypoglycemic. But, *one must be extremely careful not to ever give the alcoholic patient IV sugar prior to giving them thiamine. Administer the thiamine first* because the patient is likely to be thiamine deficient. For the sugar to be metabolized via the Kreb cycle, one needs thiamine. Whatever little bit of thiamine that may be left is going to be acutely depleted. If thiamine is not provided first, one can develop acute Wernicke's encephalopathy. With this condition, a patient will become wild, violent, and confused. Also, the patient could even die because of this simple mistake. Again, to avoid acute Wernicke's encephalopathy in alcoholics who present to the Emergency Room, treat them with thiamine first (thiamine sulfate, and then magnesium sulfate). Then, one may proceed to give the patient sugar. Start an IV that has sugar and saline in it while waiting for the results. Also, if there is difficulty in receiving the results promptly, add potassium phosphate to the IV because most alcoholics are also phosphate deficient, especially if they are vomiting. They may also become hypokalemic because they are vomiting, so one will need to also replace the potassium. It is best to replace the potassium phosphate because they may be phosphate deficient, and phosphate deficiency can cause seizures, acute confusion, and severe hemolytic anemia.

Also, it is important to do a thorough exam of the head area to make sure that there hasn't been any head injury. Remember to look inside the ears, there may be blood coming from the inner ear, and this may be the only indication that the patient has received a significant blow to the head, which may cause significant neurological problems. Also, examine the eyes, nose, mouth, and ears, very thoroughly. Perform a thorough neurological exam in order to be able to admit the patient to the hospital if necessary. When drawing the blood, always draw it for a folic acid level, and then, provide thiamine and magnesium. Next, proceed to give the patient folic acid (IM or IV) and then sugar. At this point, the patient has been provided for acutely unless there are other problems such as pneumonia or trauma. If the patient is having DT's or is being brought in because of a seizure, this must also be treated properly. Follow the same protocol that the patient cannot receive sugar until he/she receives thiamine because the seizure may be due to low blood sugar. Give the thiamine first. If the seizure is alcohol associated, the patient must be hydrated. The patient should first be treated with Phenobarbital or Valium, and once the seizure has been brought under control, proceed to make sure that the seizure was not part of a DT syndrome, because this syndrome must be handled quite differently.

The important thing to realize is that when the alcoholic presents to the Emergency Room, this individual almost always requires acute treatment, and this must be provided by someone who has experience in handling alcoholics in an Emergency Room setting.

ALCOHOLIC SEIZURES

Alcoholic seizures can be the result of acute alcohol withdrawal. They may also be due to a chronic seizure problem due to trauma to the head as the result of chronic alcohol abuse over the years. These people can have recurrent subdurals, epidurals, or other associated traumas to the brain that lead to a focus of seizures. The seizures could also be due to an electrolyte imbalance or a problem associated with vitamin deficiencies (phosphate and magnesium). Anyone of these conditions can cause acute seizures, which has to be treated appropriately.

If the patient goes into status epilepticus, he/she has to be intubated immediately to maintain a good airway. After which, they must be treated in appropriate neurological fashion and should subsequently be seen by a neurologist.

DELIRIUM TREMENS

Delirium tremens (DT's) is a condition where the patient is tremulous, confused, or has confusion deeply associated with hallucinations. These could be visual or they could be verbal, talking and not making very much sense, which may be the first or second stage or both of the DT's. Then, there is the third stage of DT's. This is when the patient is beginning to have seizures, a high fever, and is very agitated and confused. Also, the confusion is deeper as opposed to the first stage of delirium tremens. The patient now has outright DT's where he/she is seizing and elapsing into coma. A significant percentage of individuals with DT's die because of complications such as electrolyte imbalance and aspiration pneumonia. The key is to prevent the patient from going into DT's. The way one does this is, after admission to the hospital, to treat the patient orally with Librium 25 mg. four times a day (for 4–5 days) and then reduce this to twice a day. This will adequately control the individual from advancing into DT's.

If the patient is not able to take this medication by mouth, then prescribe paraldehyde and/or Ativan. Ativan is a very good medication that can be given IV. The dose is 1–2 mg. of Ativan every 6 hours. This can control the patient's agitation and prevent them from advancing into DT's. Also, the patient has to be hydrated properly. Potassium and the electrolytes have to be replaced

properly. The electrolytes have to be monitored closely. First, perform a liver profile. Then, the patient can be treated with a maintenance of thiamine 100 mg. (twice a day) and magnesium, 1 gram every day (for 4–5 days). This is sufficient to replace the magnesium store, and if they are lacking phosphate, they have to receive phosphate by (IV).

There are a lot of management problems that have to be adhered to. If the patients are infected, have sepsis, or they have pneumonia, they have to be cultured appropriately with blood cultures, sputum, urine cultures and chest x-rays. Then, they have to be treated with broad spectrum antibiotics. This is important for treating the underlying medical conditions that can complicate the problem of alcoholic associated seizures and delirium tremens.

As far as replacing vitamins, if the patient is able to take them by mouth, 1 mg. of folic acid (a day) is sufficient to replace nutritional folate deficiency. Every alcoholic who is admitted should empirically receive 1 mg of folic acid (per day) after blood is drawn for folic acid. One tablet of B complex vitamins per day should be given to replace the B complex vitamins, and 100 mg. of thiamine IM (twice a day for 4–5 days). If the patient cannot take this by mouth, then they have to be treated with IV multivitamins until they are able to do such.

TREATMENT OF ACUTE PANCREATITIS IN ALCOHOLICS

Acute pancreatitis is associated with alcohol abuse. Although pancreatitis is associated with other conditions such as gallbladder disease, alcoholism is the leading cause of pancreatitis in Blacks in this country.

Acute pancreatitis is a very serious condition. It can lead to shock and death if not recognized and treated properly. Because the pancreas secretes a tremendous amount of fluid, this fluid accumulates in the retroperitoneal area, and the alcoholic patient may come in vomiting and dehydrated. In this case, the patient has to receive large amounts of IV fluid consisting of Ringer's lactate or D5 normal saline with appropriate electrolyte replacement. This will serve to maintain the integrity of the patient's cardiovascular system. Keep them NPO (nothing by mouth) so that the pancreas can rest. Often times, one may have to put an NG tube in for appropriate nasal gastric suction. If the patient is vomiting, it is important to suction the secretions that are in the stomach to try to decrease the intensity of the vomiting. Also, appropriate antiemetics such as Compazine or Reglan can be used to control the vomiting. But, the patient will probably lose a tremendous amount of electrolytes from the vomiting, so potassium chloride or potassium phosphate must be given IV in order to replace it. Also, the patient may be febrile because of swelling of the pancreas. Sometimes he/she has to be cultured and treated with antibiotics empirically because there could be sepsis or any number of other conditions causing the fever. One cannot take the chance not to administer the patient with antibiotics.

Because acute pancreatitis is a serious condition, it has to be recognized quickly and treated with IV fluids, (keeping the patient without food), and making sure that the patient is maintained on an anabolic state by providing sugar along with sodium chloride (in the IV fluid). Acute pancreatitis has to be treated acutely and promptly to prevent death.

TREATMENT OF ACUTE
GASTRITIS IN ALCOHOLICS

The patient with acute gastritis can come in vomiting blood. It is a frequent occurrence in alcoholics because of the irritation caused by the alcohol on the wall of the stomach. Perform a gastric lavage, fluid replacement, and blood replacement to try to maintain the integrity of the cardiovascular system with the appropriate amount of blood until the patient recovers. In this setting, one has to provide H2 blockers such as Zantac IV, and Tagamet IV to try to block the secretion of acid which can intensify the gastritis.

Blacks, in this country, represent 12% of the population; Hispanics, 7%. There are 22 million people who are alcoholic in this country. Therefore, there are more people that are non-Blacks and non-Hispanic that are alcoholics; than those that are Black or Hispanic. However, more blacks drink alcohol than any other sub-group. Alcohol is a very dangerous drug. When one drinks alcohol excessively, one is likely to pay a heavy price, if not the heaviest of all, one's life. This is because of the effect that alcohol has on the total human body. There is no organ in the human anatomy that is not affected adversely by alcohol.

WHAT CAN ONE DO
TO STOP DRINKING?

Medically speaking, a patient can be treated as an outpatient by first trying them on Antabuse. This is disulfarin which is a medication that when taken causes the situation where, if one drinks, then one vomits. Not only will one vomit, but vomit in such a way that it might become lethal. Because of this one cannot take Antabuse and drink alcohol simultaneously and be comfortable.

There is another drug that one cannot take simultaneously when drinking alcohol called Flagyl. If one takes Flagyl and then drinks alcohol there is going to be an Antabuse-like reaction, that can be very severe and at times, also fatal. If the patient needs psychiatric help, he/she can go to a therapist that has experience in dealing with alcoholism, and, hopefully, they will receive help.

While the patient is withdrawing from alcohol addiction in the hospital as well as an outpatient setting, it is important to give the patient some other medication such as Librium to take the edge off the anxiety and nervousness. This anxiety is associated with not drinking alcohol after one has been drinking for a long time and then stops. Also, this prevents the patient from going into delirium tremens. Again, it is important to make sure one treats the patient with Librium while they withdraw from drinking.

It is important to stress the fact that Librium and alcohol cannot be taken together. This is a lethal combination. Alcohol, a neurosuppressant, and Librium, a combination of the two, can lead to coma and death. If the patient is alcoholic and is to be treated with some type of anti-anxiety medication, *it has to be clear that they cannot drink alcohol*. The purpose of the anti-anxiety medication is to reduce anxiety while they are withdrawing from the alcohol. After withdrawal, it is medically proper to give them anyone of these anti-anxiety medications: Librium, Valium, Ativan, or Xanax. Anyone of these will work to reduce the anxiety until the patient can become completely independent of any of these substances. It is a good idea to go to a psychiatrist, clinic, or private doctor and get involved in an anti-alcohol-drinking organization. Most of these are very well organized, and they know how to help one to stop drinking on a long-term basis.

It is very important to realize that once an alcoholic, always an alcoholic, just like once a drug addict, always a drug addict. This does not mean that one is always using drugs or drinking alcohol, but the personality trait that led to the addiction is still present. Therefore, one has to make a lifetime commitment to the whole concept of not abusing alcohol in order to fully recover.

UNDERLYING PSYCHIATRIC PROBLEMS IN ALCOHOLICS

A lot of individuals who are alcoholics have underlying psychiatric problems to begin with, and sometimes these underlying psychiatric problems play a major role as to why the person is drinking. In fact, alcoholics commit suicide 30–40 times more than the general population. This is why it is always important that the individual seeks some form of psychiatric help to try to deal with the possibility that he/she may indeed have underlying problems that need to be dealt with.

FETAL ALCOHOL SYNDROME

Alcoholism during pregnancy is dangerous. Up to 5,000 babies per year are affected by fetal alcohol syndrome. More specifically, 1 in close to 800 babies that are born are affected with the fetal alcohol syndrome, leading to all sorts of birth defects and mental retardation. Approximately, 36–37,000 newborn babies each year are affected by the wide range of alcohol associated birth problems, and approximately 2–3 births per 1,000 are affected by some form of alcohol associated problems.

For every 1,000 births that occur in the black community, 10 babies die because of a whole host of alcohol associated problems.

But, even more devastating than fetal alcohol syndrome alone is the fact that some mothers drink and take a whole lot of other drugs, causing their babies to die. The United States is one of the richest countries of the world, yet 19 babies die for every 1,000 births in the black community. It is less than half this number in the white community where 9 babies per 1,000 births will die.

This is a catastrophe because these pregnant women either do not receive or do not seek any prenatal care. Therefore, when they do present for delivery, they have a whole host of medical problems such as pre-eclampsia and eclampsia. Both baby and mother are often anemic; the mother may also be diabetic. Babies born to mothers with these conditions are likely to be born prematurely and or develop a whole host of other serious medical problems decreasing their chances of surviving the peri-natal period.

SEXUAL DYSFUNCTION AS A RESULT OF ALCOHOL ABUSE

As far as sexual function is concerned, some individuals drink to heighten their sexual capabilities prior to sexual intercourse. This is a transient phenomenon because when one drinks alcohol chronically there is definitely a decrease in libido both in women and men. It is a hormonal malfunction because there is an excess in estrogen production. This excess is because the liver is damaged by the alcohol to a degree where it is unable to break down estrogen. If a woman has too much estrogen, she may overstimulate the endometrium and may develop breakthrough vaginal bleeding. Her desire for sex decreases because there is an abnormality in the function of the nerves that are necessary to stimulate sexual arousal. In the man, the situation is worse because the man may not be able to have an erection. In order for a man to have an erection, there has to be a combination of blood flow plus good nerve stimulation. When the nerves are damaged by the effect of alcohol, it creates a problem for proper sexual functioning in both men and women.

In addition to this, an increased level of estrogen in the man, as mentioned, may cause gynecomastia (enlarged breasts) and decrease in the size of the glans penis and also causes shiny skin of the testicles. This is the effect of too much estrogen. Also, the inability of the liver to break down estrogen causes the man to have a decrease in libido because the estrogen competes with the androgen resulting in decrease of sexual desire,

decrease in the size of the glans penis, and in all sorts of other sexual aberrations. All of these problems are the result of the inability of alcohol damaged liver to break down estrogen. Since men and women both have adrenal glands, this is another mechanism through which estrogen can be produced from fat cells leading to a further elevation of estrogen in the blood stream and more estrogen associated alcoholic liver disease side effects to the genital organs.

ALCOHOL ABUSE AND ABUSE OF PRESCRIPTION DRUGS

Another issue to be discussed is the whole concept of alcohol abuse and the abuse of prescription drugs such as Valium, Librium, Xanax, Ativan and a whole host of other sedatives. Individuals who drink alcohol tend to use alcohol and also use these drugs because they have a summation effect. Alcohol is a neurological suppressant, a respiratory suppressant, and a cardiac suppressant. These drugs also have neurological suppressant effects, and cardiac depressive effects, and respiratory depressive effects. When an individual abuses alcohol and also abuses sedatives, he/she might develop the summation effect that can lead to respiratory arrest which can lead to cardiac arrest. This can lead to coma, total anesthesia, and death. So, it is not only dangerous for one to abuse alcohol, but it is also dangerous to abuse sedatives and may be even fatal to abuse a combination of both. This is a formula for disaster which can only lead to death.

METHADONE AND ALCOHOL

Individuals who are former drug abusers and are trying to stop using heroin or cocaine and are on Methadone usually use alcohol as a means of becoming less tense and less agitated. Hence, there is a large population of former heroin addicts who are now on Methadone who abuse alcohol excessively as a means of substitution. Again, that is a formula for catastrophe because Methadone, (although it is supposed to be less addicting than heroin) is also an addicting medication and when combined with alcohol, it can be lethal.

YEARLY DEATH RATE DUE TO ALCOHOL ASSOCIATED CIRRHOSIS OF THE LIVER

Cirrhosis of the liver accounts for close to 40,000 deaths per year according to published reports. Cirrhosis also has associated medical problems that can lead to death. *The leading cause of death from alcohol abuse is cirrhosis of the liver, and its associated problems and infections.*

Infection occurs because alcoholism affects the immune system and white cells are decreased. Even if these cells are normal in number, they become malfunctioning. However, to make the situation worse, leukopenia (low white blood cell count) is frequently associated with alcoholism. Because of the cirrhosis of the liver which results in hypersplenism (an enlarged spleen), this also causes the destruction of the white cells. There exists two problems with the white cells: 1. They are not functioning properly from an immune deficiency standpoint. 2. The number of white cells are less because of the fact that the spleen is enlarged, and the enlargement of the spleen is causing the destruction of white cells inappropriately. So, infection becomes very common.

In addition to this, as mentioned, when the individuals are drunk, they lose their swallowing reflexes, and they tend to aspirate leading to aspiration pneumonia and lung abscesses that are extremely difficult to treat medically. Very frequently, these individuals succumb to sepsis or adult respiratory distress syndrome, ventilatory failure, and to death. So, pulmonary deaths are the result of infections that are resistant to antibiotics.

This is partly because the overall anatomy is weakened because the individual is so malnourished and debilitated by the effects of alcohol. And thus, they succumb to infection.

In spite of the tremendous amounts of very powerful antibiotics, modern medicine is still losing these people. Because of the fact that their condition is so poor, they do not always respond to treatment.

The second most common cause of death related to alcoholism is bleeding secondary to cirrhosis of the liver. Even though there is the ability to transfuse blood, plasma, platelets, and other associated blood components, these individuals are being lost because often the bleeding is so extensive and severe. For instance, bleeding may occur because of varices. Variceal bleeding is very difficult in an acute setting to stop. Namely, the individuals (because of the obstruction of normal circulation within the liver) have increased pressure and the portal system is obstructed. This is portal hypertension. Then, they may develop neovascularization with small little vessels superficially growing on the surface of the upper GI tract, especially in the esophageal area. When these vessels rupture because of vomiting and retching, it causes a bleeding problem. Once it starts, it is very difficult to stop. One may need to have a gastroenterologist endoscope the patient to identify the problem. Also, there is a procedure whereby the individual is made to swallow a balloon that becomes inflated to put pressure on those vessels to stop bleeding. It is a very horrifying procedure because they are aspirating blood. It is a terrible situation to watch when somebody is exsanguinating from variceal bleeding. Treatment options of variceal bleeding include IV Pritressin, Cryo treatment with laser and Inderal treatment to lower the portal pressure.

These things work transiently in some individuals, but by and large, they do not always work. Variceal bleeding is a dangerous type of problem, and it usually results in dealth.

They can bleed excessively, resulting in hypotension, which in turn can lead to cardiac arrest. They are in no condition to be taken to the Operating Room because this type of bleeding cannot be stopped by any operation. In the past, to deal with the variceal bleeding problem, some shunt procedures were tried, i.e., Hepato renal shunt. These almost uniformly ended in disasters with the patient becoming encephalopathic and dying. There is no real surgical procedure of any value that can be performed to stop this kind of bleeding. The important thing is for one not to develop varices to begin with. Once one has developed them, they can start bleeding at any moment and this can lead to death.

A major problem associated with G.I. bleeding in alcoholics is the deposition of blood within the G.I. tracts. Because the blood contains a tremendous amount of protein, (Blood in fact is nothing but protein), it gets acted upon by the bacteria in the gut. Then, it passes into the urea pathway, the urea cycle, and generates ammonia. The ammonia becomes reabsorbed. Ammonia is toxic to the brain. Therefore, once the ammonia is reabsorbed a cycle develops, where one cannot metabolize ammonia properly, resulting in encephalopathy leading to coma, seizures, and death. Sometimes, alcoholics are given lactulose, which is a diarrhea inducing medication that can prevent them from reabsorbing the blood by preventing the blood from being broken down. And, they are constantly having bloody diarrhea to prevent the protein from being absorbed. Most of the time, they cannot take this by mouth because they have to be kept on NPO (nothing by mouth). Lactulose can be given through a nasal gastric tube. By and large, they develop liver failure with a hepatorenal syndrome leading to all types of electrolyte imbalances. Most often, alcoholics who may be in the best of hands and under the best of circumstances die from the toxicity. All this is the result of alcohol abuse secondary to cirrhosis of the liver. This condition eventually leads to bleeding which can lead to encephalopathy; and this eventually leads to complications and death.

ACUTE ALCOHOL TOXICITY ON PLATELETS

Alcohol, itself, is acutely toxic to platelets. Any large amount of alcohol consumption can cause one's platelet count to decrease because this may actually develop into bone marrow failure. Bone marrow failure is the failure to produce red cells, white cells, and platelets because of acute alcohol abuse. Again, chronic alcohol abuse can cause chronic liver problems, leading to portal hypertension, and leading to hypersplenism.

HYPERSPLENISM AND ITS CLINICAL MANIFESTATIONS; COMPLICATIONS AS A RESULT OF ALCOHOL ABUSE

Once one has an enlarged spleen, there is going to be a decrease in platelets, a decrease in red cells, a decrease in white cells or any combination of these three cells can become low. The low red cells occur because of bone marrow failure and or hemolysis. Once one is hemolyzing, there is a breaking up of red cells. To transfuse these individuals with blood, one must also deal with all the complications of blood transfusions which include: hepatitis B, hepatitis C, cytomegalovirus infection, and the HIV-I virus leading to AIDS. Today, blood transfusions and blood component transfusions are associated with a whole host of problems that can ultimately lead to the patient's death if they become infected with any one of these listed viruses.

DIFFERENT TYPES OF ALCOHOL RELATED BLEEDING PROBLEMS

It is very important to be able to acutely differentiate the bleeding that occurs in an alcoholic. The alcoholic individual generally has severe liver disease as the result of alcohol abuse. This same individual may present to the Emergency Room bleeding acutely and one must ask is it due to liver failure or is it due to DIC (disseminated intravascular coagulopathy)? This is crucial to differentiate because the approach to these two problems are so very different.

In liver disease one will expect the prothrombin time to be high but the prothrombin time will also be high in DIC. So, in liver disease one will see a prolonged prothrombin time, a prolonged factor VII, Factor IX, and factor X because those are the so-called vitamin K dependent factors, II, VII, IX and X. These factors are all made in the liver.

In DIC on the other hand, expect to have an elevation in Factor II which causes the prothrombin time to be increased. Also, there is going to be decreased fibrinogen which is Factor I in addition to a low platelet count. However, low platelet counts can also be seen in liver disease so that is the reason why it is important to differentiate between DIC and liver failure leading to coagulopathy. In liver failure leading to coagulopathy, the *fibrinogen is expected to be normal,* but in DIC *the fibrinogen is almost always low.*

One must look at the peripheral smear and should see a low platelet on the smear. Usually, the peripheral blood smear will have anywhere from 8–15 platelets p/hpf. On the other hand, if one has thrombocytopenia (which is low platelets) one may see only 1 or 2 platelets or none at all p/hpf, and if one is dealing with DIC one may see schistocytes (red cells that are fragmented with little spindle-like structures and a little thread-like material). The cell is being eroded by the spleen, and one is seeing pieces of red cells that are left. One might also see helmet cells. One sees this also in DIC. If one sees schistocytes, helmet cells and a low platelet count on the smear, this is consistent with DIC. But, one has to be very careful that the smear is not taken from the finger. If one takes a smear from someone's finger, the platelets aggregate so fast that it is going to appear to be low on the smear. It is important to obtain the smear from a tube of blood that has the EDTA in it, (the lavender tube). It is very important from a technical point because when the platelets appear to be low on the smear, one has to ask the question of how the smear was made. Was it made from the finger stick or was it made from blood taken from the lavender tube which has EDTA in it? If it is taken from the lavender tube, this is an accurate reflection of the platelet count. But, if it is taken from the finger and then smeared and appears to be low, then it is not an accurate reflection. It may not be low at all. These are crucial important points that have to be kept in mind when one is trying to make a decision as to what is wrong with the patient in regards to bleeding.

Coagulopathy Due to Liver Disease

It is very important that DIC be differentiated from coagulopathy due to liver disease because in coagulopathy (due to liver disease), one can attempt to give the patient an injection of Vitamin K. If the prothrombin time is high and the platelets are very low, it is wise to give the injection in the deltoid. In the deltoid, one can apply pressure to prevent bleeding. If it is given in the thigh or buttocks, one may induce severe bleeding that can result in a large hematoma that can become very problematic. However, Vitamin K 10–15 mg. given IM will take from 6–12 hours to reverse the abnormal coagulopathy if it is due to Vitamin K deficiency. On the other hand, if one has to move promptly to correct the abnormality, it is best that one infuse the patient with fresh frozen plasma. If one gives fresh frozen plasma, the whole problem can be corrected anywhere from 2–4 hours after infusion because one is actually replacing factors that are missing. Fresh frozen plasma contains all these factors that are low because of liver failure such as factor II, VII, and IX.

On the other hand, in DIC one should be equipped to perform the 5 and 10 test immediately. This is another way of differentiating the problem. Factor X is always low in liver failure but it is normal in DIC. Factor V is normal in liver failure, but it is low in DIC. These are the ways one can differentiate abnormal liver function tests due to liver failure from DIC (disseminated intravascular coagulopathy) which is important because DIC has no specific treatments. In DIC, one really has to treat the underlying condition. If it is sepsis or shock, treat it. If it is cancer, provide treatment for the cancer and by bringing the cancer under control, hopefully the DIC will be controlled. But, sometimes, this does not happen. There are certain conditions such as acute myelocytic leukemia that have a propensity to present as DIC, especially acute promyelocytic leukemia. If the patient is bleeding from the gums and bleeding from every orifice, it may be that the patient has acute leukemia with DIC accompanying the problem.

If the patient has liver failure, the treatment is factor replacement. Replace platelets and replace the coagulation factors by giving fresh frozen plasma. Giving IM Vitamin K in this setting is a clinical manipulation that allows the physician to determine how much good liver the patient has left. If the patient corrects the prothrombin time by receiving Vitamin K, this is a good indication that this particular patient may have some very healthy liver left over. If the liver is severely damaged, it would not be able to synthesize (produce) the coagulation factors that it normally produces; therefore, when Vitamin K is given, the prothrombin time (PT) will not be corrected toward normal. But, if it does, that means then the liver still has reserve, and if alcohol is refrained from, there may be a chance for recovery of the liver function.

Bleeding is one of the ways that people die from alcohol abuse. Infection, as stated above, is another way. The key is when bleeding is taking place, immediately seek the advice of a hematologist (an expert in the field of coagulopathy and bleeding disorders). But it is not every time that when a patient comes in bleeding, it is due to gastritis or to an ulcer. It may be indeed due to a coagulopathy which manifests itself as vomiting of blood, etc. It is important to have a good understanding of the pathophysiology of the bleeding from alcoholism since it is probably *the number one cause of death.*

Another way that patients with acute alcoholic intoxication (an alcohol level of over 400 mg. per ml), can result in coma and death is because of seizures. If seizures are not treated appropriately, they can develop into a situation where one can die from status epilepticus. The patient can die of asphyxiation because when he/she is seizing, there is an inability to breathe, because the airway is compromised. If status epilepticus develops, the patient should be intubated so that the airway can be controlled and appropriate oxygen can be administered to prevent the patient from dying from anoxia. This is one way acute seizures can lead to death. Also, acute seizures have other complications. If the patient is seizing, and there is no one around to control his/her tongue by putting a tongue depressor or other device in the mouth, the patient can bite his/her tongue so violently that one can bleed and choke on his/her own tongue. The patient may also develop delirium tremens.

DIFFERENT STAGES OF DELIRIUM TREMENS

As stated previously, delirium tremens have several stages and in its final stage, the deeper stage, (when the patient is really comatose and seizing), the patient can actually die. A significant percentage of patients with delirium tremens die regardless of the treatment provided for them. Neurological death does occur as a result of acute alcoholism.

Delirium tremens usually develops anywhere from 72 hours after a person stops drinking, and sometimes, 4–5 days, or even a week later. Whenever a patient who has a history of heavy alcohol abuse is admitted, immediately one has to write an order to watch closely for the possibility of the development of DT's. Also, the patient has to be given medications such as Librium to prevent DT's from developing. When it develops, it is not always easy to revert it. Proper hydration and proper electrolyte replacement is crucial to maintain the patient in a good electrolyte balance and a good anabolic stage. This is done so that the patient can recover in time with the appropriate maintenance of medical care. If this is not done, the patient is going to die as a result of DT's (another acute way of dying from the effects of alcoholism).

DEADLY CONSEQUENCES OF ALCOHOL ABUSE

It can cause tremendous damage to the persons who drink excessively and the chances of recovery sometimes are nil if the patient is not in a setting where appropriate medical care can be administered. Unfortunately, for Blacks who almost always end up in city hospitals where the care most of the time is suboptimal. This is due to a variety of reasons: lack of staff, lack of experienced physicians, lack of nursing experience, and lack of enough nurses to watch the patients and take care of them. This is one of the rea-

sons why the death rate among Blacks and other minorities who suffer from alcoholism and its multitude of complications are so much higher than the white counterparts. Blacks and other minorities receive their medical care in facilities that are not well equipped to provide the necessary care. Sometimes, they end up sitting in the Emergency Room setting (anywhere from 6–12 hours waiting to be seen) while they are dehydrated, hungry, and hypoglycemic (because they have not eaten substantially for so very long). Only when they start seizing or something acute develops, that they receive care and frequently the damage has already occurred.

PSYCHOLOGICAL PROBLEMS OF ALCOHOLISM AND THEIR DESTRUCTIVE IMPACT ON BLACK FAMILIES AND THE BLACK COMMUNITY

Alcoholism is always devastating to the family and particularly to the black family. It can cause a great deal of suffering. Because black individuals are under stress from bigotry, and racism, they resort to alcohol to try and ease the pain. They do not realize that, in fact, alcohol is a drug that is killing them. It causes a lot of pain to the family, and it can kill other people through vehicular accidents and homicides. In the black community, greater than 90% of the victims of murder are killed by other blacks that live in the same community. If Blacks are going to be victimized, they are more likely to be victimized by other Blacks living in the same community. Blacks kill Blacks more than Whites kill Blacks. It is a vicious cycle. When people are angry and drunk, they turn on each other with knives and guns. Something has to be done to decrease the incidence of alcohol abuse in the Black community. It is important that the Black community strive to overcome all of the associated problems of alcoholism. The overall health of the Black community is in a shamble presently. And, the death rate is very high because of alcohol-related problems. As stated earlier, close to 40,000 people per year are dying as a result of cirrhosis. There are a host of other problems, leading to death associated with alcohol. Such as vehicular accidents, homicides, and pneumonia. Alcohol abuse can also lead to death from pneumonia. Acute GI bleeding resulting from gastritis is associated with alcoholism. Death from chronic pancreatitis is real. Death from alcoholic associated heart disease is quite high. In order to improve the Black community, Blacks have to be made aware of the devastation that alcohol abuse can cause, and to stop abusing alcohol, period.

DIFFERENT ORGANIZATIONS THAT ARE INVOLVED IN HELPING PEOPLE TO STOP DRINKING ALCOHOL

There are a whole host of organizations in this country that are set up such as A.A. to try to help individuals to stop drinking. A.A. is a world wide organization to help people who have a problem with drinking alcohol.

It is recommended that the Blacks, and other minorities who have problems with alcohol abuse should contact these organizations, so, that they can hopefully get the help they need in order to stop drinking.

There are a whole host of Black organizations that are set up to help people who have a drinking problem. As it relates to the Black community, there is the National Black Alcoholism Council. This is an organization organized in 1978 to help Black people with alcohol problems. Also, there is the Institute on Black Chemical Abuse. There is the National Coalition of Hispanic Health and

Human Resources; to help Hispanics who have drinking problems. Also, there are the Hispanic Health Council and National Hispanic Family Against Drug Abuse.

Also, there is the National Association of Native American Children of Alcoholics. And, the National Asian Family Against Substance Abuse, in addition. All of these organizations are in action and are there to help people who have problems with alcohol regardless of race.

CONCLUSION

Because Blacks are mostly poor, they are under much more pressure. Since alcohol is cheap and easy to buy, Blacks buy it because it is a cheap escape, but they are killing themselves with it. Also, they are not only killing themselves but they are destroying their families, and a significant percentage of other members of the society (crimes), (vehicular accidents). They are causing their families misery by being irresponsible, breaking marital relationships. Also, black alcoholics become unemployed and unemployable because they are so disabled because of the effect of alcohol. Their families wind up on welfare. And, a significant proportion of them become homeless because they lose their jobs. Associated with the alcohol abuse is a whole host of other high risk behavior such as illicit drug abuse and involvement with prostitutes leading to the contraction of the HIV, Type I virus that can lead to AIDS, etc.

The best one can hope for is that the black community will begin to look after itself. It must try to learn the best way to avoid these outrageous conditions so that Blacks can lead a better and healthier life. If it does not do this, then there is no positive future for the Black community as it exists presently.

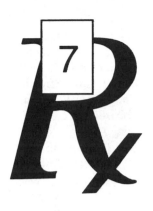

DRUG ADDICTION AND ITS ASSOCIATED PROBLEMS IN AFRICAN-AMERICANS

CHAPTER OUTLINE

INCIDENCE OF DRUG ADDICTION

According to the latest estimates, there are about 2 to 2-1/2 million Heroin addicts in the United States. Of these, some 70 to 75% are African-American. Also, there are about a million or more cocaine addicts, and more than 3-1/2 million marijuana addicts. In this country, there are several million more individuals who are drug dependent.

The total cost to the American economy because of drug addiction is estimated between 33–36 million dollars a year. This involves loss of work, health care services, crimes, and accidents associated with drug use.

Drugs like PCP and LSD are also becoming a major problem in terms of addiction.

Now, there is a new form of drug called "crack cocaine". This is a more powerful form of cocaine, and its effects are much more devastating than cocaine. It takes only between 3 weeks to 2 months for someone to become addicted to "crack cocaine". Because it is cheap, ($10.00) it is a favorite drug for teen-agers, and they become addicted to it. Crack-cocaine streamlines into the blood and brain quickly. Individuals who use crack become completely vicious. There is nothing under the sun that they will not do when they are addicted. They will even kill to supply their addiction.

In the early 60's, Heroin was the common street drug. Cocaine was expensive and really for the middle and upper class. Now, cocaine, in the crack form of it, is not expensive. It is no longer just a drug for the upper and middle class, but has extended to the lower class.

TYPES OF ADDICTING PRESCRIPTION DRUGS

Besides street drugs, it is also important to mention prescription drugs that are abused. They are: Opium, Codeine, and Mor-phine. Also, the barbituates. They consist of Quaaludes, Placidyl, and Doridin. And, stimulant type drugs (amphetamines) such as Dexedrine, and Diphetamine and Biphetamine, Eqanil, Miltown, Dilaudid, Percodan, Demerol, Darvon, Talwin, Darvocet; the barbituates such as Phenobarbital, Nembutal, Seconal, Tuanil, Pentothal, Amytol, Restoril, Halcion, Dalmane, Zanax, Ativan, Librium, Valium, and Tranxene. All these drugs are abused. These are the prescription drugs talked about. *Some doctors over-prescribe these addicting drugs and contribute indirectly to the addiction that is running rampant in our society.*

HEROIN ADDICTION

Heroin is administered intravenously, and because of this, there are many complications. There develops a psychological dependence of the drug because the brain becomes accustomed to it, and if it is not available, a craving develops. This craving can become so severe that the individual will do anything including (stealing, mugging, and killing) to obtain money to buy the drug. This is what is called "the conditioning phenomena". However, as mentioned there are other problems because it is administered intravenously. Often, the needles are infected with hepatitis B and hepatitis non-A and non-B. Also, cytomegalovirus and the AIDS virus can be transmitted intravenously. Hence, there is a very high incidence of the AIDS virus in the IV drug addicted population. Also, syphilis and other bacterial infections such as staphylococcus infections, strep infections and other gram negative organisms such as pseudomonas, and also fungal infections, can be transmitted intravenously. As a matter of fact, malaria can also be transmitted by this means. Bacterial organism that is transmitted through dirty needles can cause endocarditis, (either acute bacterial endocarditis or subacute bacterial endocarditis) leading to the erosion of the heart valves which can lead to heart failure, arrhythmias, and death. This can also lead to septic emboli to the lung, and brain abscesses (as the result of septic emboli to the brain) and to an infection of the kidneys, and other parts of the body. So, the infections associated with IV drug abuse can be devastating and frequently leads to the death of the individual.

INTRAVENOUS DRUG ABUSE AND CARDIAC INFECTION: ACUTE VS. SUBACUTE BACTERIAL ENDOCARDITIS

Bacteria that is found in the needles (because the needle is not sterilized), finds its way into the blood stream. From the blood stream, it passes into the right side of the heart and settles on the different heart valves, the aortic valve, the mitral valves, or the tricuspid valves. It basically erodes the valves away, and then sometimes the vegetation that settled on the valve of the heart gets dispersed into the rest of the body as septic emboli to the lungs, to the brain, leading to lung abscesses and brain abscesses. Even abscesses to the kidneys can occur. These individuals sometimes develop congestive heart failure complicated with all sorts of cardiac arrhythmias because of endocarditis. IV drug abusers have a tendency to develop gram positive subacute bacterial endocarditis or acute bacterial carditis. They are infected by the staphylococci, streptococci, strep bovis, gram negative organisms, fungi of different kinds. Now, they are being infected with AIDS because AIDS is transmitted via the blood, also. Once the needle is infected (it has the HIV type I virus on it) and they exchange needles—they transmit the HIV Type I virus to each other.

With Heroin addiction, when one begins to crave it, they can experience a withdrawal. The withdrawal can cause severe seizures,—during an acute seizure the individual may die.

Another condition, (not only the overdose of Heroin) occurs with the individuals presenting with pinpoint pupils, not breathing, and are in a coma. Treatment is to give Narcan IV to revert the effect of the Heroin. If they present with pinpoint pupils, cannot breathe, and have needle tracks in the arm, they have to receive Narcan (also known as Naloxone). They usually get a first dose and then a Narcan drip to try to revert the effect of the Heroin.

METHADONE

Methadone is a medication that is given as a substitute for Heroin in an attempt to get the individual off the Heroin. They are placed into a Methadone program, (The Methadone maintenance program), where it is administered in liquid form. But, Methadone can also kill. If one takes an overdose of Methadone the effect is similar to an overdose of Heroin. Pinpoint pupils, shallow respiration, tachycardia with rapid death—if Narcan is not given immediately to revert the effects. Frequently these individuals have to be intubated in order to breathe while the Narcan is being administered in order to try to revert the overdose.

Also in dealing with both Methadone and Heroin addicts, these individuals can come into the hospital with pulmonary edema (fluid in the lung), one of the side effects of the Heroin and Methadone.

COCAINE

There is cocaine hydrochloride powder that is injected or inhaled. There is cocaine alkaloid which is free based, and "crack" that is smoked. All these things have different strength and ability to intoxicate the individual. And, then cause all sorts of serious problems. Some of the signs of intoxication of cocaine include tachycardia, pupillary dilatation. The blood pressure may be increased. There may also be fever, chills, vomiting, visual hallucination, euphoria and impaired judgment, and a feeling that insects are crawling on the skin. Also, there is a whole fluctuation of moods (increased sexual interest) which deal with anxiety, craving for the cocaine, fatigue and irritability. This may last anywhere from 24–48 hours. The important thing is to realize that if they don't have appropriate medication, they can go into withdrawal. Withdrawal can occur anywhere from 24 hours off the drug and can lead to seizures, severe depression, and cocaine deliriums. Associated with this can be violence whereby patients have to be restrained.

Acute Cardiac Decompensation

Acute cardiac decompensation is another problem associated with cocaine. These people can develop severe cardiac arrhythmia. They can develop spasm of the coronary arteries leading to acute myocardial infarction and sudden death. There is an acute component to the problem of cocaine withdrawal which can lead to cardiac arrest. Also, a cocaine overdose if not treated properly, can lead to respiratory and cardiac problems that can also lead to death.

OPIOIDS

Opioid Toxicities

The opioids are a family of drugs including: Heroin, Codeine, Meperidine, Hydromorphone and Oxycodone.

Sometimes addicts use needles subcutaneously because they have poor veins and they can't get into a vein. This is another source of bacteria entering into the blood stream leading to endocarditis, sepsis resulting in death of these individuals secondary to decompensation of the heart.

The syndrome of Heroin induced pulmonary edema is an acute entity. Patients who present to the emergency room with this problem must be treated immediately with IV Narcan and frequently these patients must be intubated to allow time for Narcan to take effect. Patients must also be treated with standard medications such as oxygen and IV diuretics.

One of the many problems the health team may run into when treating a patient with a narcotic overdose is that the patient may have no good veins to administer medication such as Narcan. In these situations, sometimes a cut down of the arm or leg may be necessary to get an access to start these intravenous medications. These individuals have basically given up on life and they just self destroy themselves. By the time they present themselves to a doctor in an emergency room setting, they are extremely sick. They have all sorts of medical complications. They are poorly kept and overall they have poor hygiene. But, they are human beings, and they are patients, and they have rights. They are entitled to the best medical care that medicine can offer and they should receive this care.

If a person is a heroin addict and if he or she wants to give up the habit of using heroin he or she can join a methadone program. Methadone can be taken once a day as a substitute for heroin. Unfortunately, a great deal of the time the subgroup of these individuals are involved in selling the Methadone. Sometimes they drink the methadone, and they regurgitate it as soon as they get out of the door and sell it in the street. This is why programs don't prescribe tablets of methadone because it would be easier to sell the tablets. These individuals also have the problem of substituting. Since the methadone is not sufficient, in most cases, to allow them to crush the urge of the Heroin that they have been using, they couple methadone with alcohol or any other type of drugs that they can obtain.

PREGNANCY AND DRUG ADDICTION

Another tragic situation that exists for Heroin addicts is the woman who is a Heroin addict and becomes pregnant. If she continues to use Heroin while she is pregnant, she is going to give birth to a baby who is going to be markedly affected by the effect of the Heroin. The baby may be born prematurely, malnourished, or with a whole host of birth defects. And, the baby is born withdrawing from Heroin, and may have seizures and other psychomotor abnormalities. For one thing, most Heroin addicted infants are born with a low Apgar. The Apgar is a scale that is used to determine how well the baby is doing in the first few minutes of birth. A low Apgar (of 4–5) indicates that there may be oxygen delivery impairment to the brain which may in the future lead to learning difficulty. (A good Apgar is an Apgar of 8–9.) Once the baby's cardiac and respiratory systems are suppressed and depressed by the effect of the Heroin, this directly results in a low Apgar. In addition to having difficulty during utero, when the baby is born, there is often great difficulty in getting the infant to take a first breath to allow oxygen into the brain (often a very immature and premature brain). Lack of proper amount of oxygen to the brain of the fetus or the newly born baby can cause permanent brain damage. Often times, one wonders why it is that these children cannot learn in school as they appear to be physically normal. One has to examine the condition under which the children were born. If they were born under a condition where the mother was addicted to Heroin, the child was born with a respiratory system and a cardiovascular system that was depressed. This causes the inability of the blood to be shunted to the brain leading to brain damage with possible epileptic seizures and a whole host of other chronic abnormalities that appear later on in life.

So, drug addiction does not only affect the father, does not only affect the mother; it affects frequently the baby, who is the innocent part of the whole setting. And, the baby goes on to suffer for life if he/she survives into adulthood, because he/she was born into a subculture where he/she was affected by drug from the time they are in utero. No wonder these children become slow learners. How can they learn, when they have brains that were damaged from the time they were in the mother's womb?

HALLUCINOGENS AND THEIR TOXICITIES

Hallucinogens have their own problems. The hallucinogens are very common among the college crowd and basically come into the category of LSD (acid diethylamide), and DMT, Dimethyltriptamine and Mescaline. These different drugs can manifest themselves by behavior aberration, depression, anxiety, fear of losing one's mind, and paranoia. Then, there are some of the physical findings such as sweating, tachycardia, palpitation, blurring of vision, tremors, incoordination, auricular fibrillation, dilatation, and personality disorders. These are very serious problems. If these drugs are used for a long period of time, they can damage one's mind chronically.

AMPHETAMINES: ADDICTIVE POTENTIALS AND THEIR TOXICITIES

Amphetamines are very common among the college type groups. PCP (Phencyclidine) are taken in school in order to try to stay awake so one can study. Then one develops a desire to have them all the time. They also cause grandiose psychomotor agitation, impaired judgment, impaired social and intellectual function and hypervigilance. Physical signs are: elevated blood pressure, nausea, vomiting, tachycardia. These are some of the symptoms of this problem. Eventually, this condition leads to chronic psychosis. All these conditions are very damaging to the brain because the brain is very sensitive, and was not meant to deal with this condition.

SEDATIVES: HYPNOTICS, ADDICTIVE POTENTIALS AND THEIR TOXICITIES

Drugs such as benzodiazapine, flurazepam, glutethimide, chloral hydrate, metaquinone, barbiturates are prescribed medication (and over-prescribed by some doctors) and are addicting. Sometimes they are coupled with alcohol and literally can kill by taking too much and also drinking alcohol at the same time. What is the mind set that leads someone to get involved with these medications while other individuals are able to withstand the pressures of life and refrain from getting involved with these addicting substances. Individuals who become addicted to addicting drugs and alcohol usually have underlying psychological problems that make them fall under the influence of these addicting substances. They feel that drugs strengthens their ability to function under pressure, and that is a wrong and dangerous concept which must be avoided at all cost. Sometimes these individuals come from families where there is a high incidence of addiction to drugs and alcohol.

DRUG ADDICTION AND MEDICAL PROBLEMS

Drug addiction is a multisystem disease. The drug gets into the blood stream and the blood goes everywhere in the body. Therefore, there is hardly any organ in the body that would not be affected in some fashion by drugs within the blood.

EFFECTS OF DRUG ADDICTION ON THE BRAIN

With the brain there are psychological abnormalities, dependency on the brain and evidence that there could be degeneration in the brain tissue leading to dementia. Chronic drug dementia is when there is a lack of ability to concentrate, loss of memory, and seizure disorders.

INFECTIONS ASSOCIATED WITH IV DRUG ADDICTION

Another common infection that the IV drug abusers get is hepatitis B or hepatitis Non A or Non B which can lead to a multitude of acute complications secondary to liver problems. In this type of infection the individual can develop jaundice acutely, becomes fabrile, has loss of appetite and loss of taste for cigarettes. There may be low platelet count, associated with coagulopathy due to high prothombin time, high partial thromboplastin time; all because of liver failure secondary to the effect of the hepatitis on the liver. The sum total of all these problems is bleeding complications.

If the person has had hepatitis for a while, then cirrhosis of the liver may develop which may lead to portal hypertension leading to hypersplenism and pancytopenia with hemolysis.

These individuals can go on to develop liver decompensation with ascites secondary to hyperaldosteronism leading to salt retention and fluid retention with massive edema in the legs and abdomen (which is very difficult to mobilize). Also, they can have spontaneous peritonitis which is where the bowel leaks stool into the cavity of the abdomen. They can have a tense and painful abdomen and if taken to the OR in such weak and sick condition, this is a formula for catastrophe. The best approach is to treat with IV antibiotic until the situation quiets down.

There is a high incidence of syphilis in the IVDA population because syphilis is transmitted both via blood and also sexually. A significant percentage of the IVDA sub-population become prostitutes, selling their sexual favors in order to find money to buy drugs. They become infected with gonorrhea and non-gonorrheal urethritis, chlamydia, and they also develop herpes. There is a high incidence of herpes infections in the drug addict population because it is a sexually transmitted disease. Of course, the most devastating of all is AIDS. So 75% of the IV drug abusers in New York City (of which there are close to 600,000) are said to be infected with the HIV virus. Groups such as these place the heterosexual community in the greatest danger of being infected with AIDS. IV drug abuse is a devastating medical problem which costs billions every year. More people are using drugs, and more and more drugs are finding their way into the Black community.

COCAINE ADDICTIONS

If cocaine is used IV then one really runs into the same complications that one sees in Heroin, such as sepsis, and all the complications of sepsis such as endocarditis. On the other hand, those who use the nasal passage for the purpose of snorting cocaine often times develop nosebleeds and the nasal septum is destroyed, creating holes in the nasal septum because of the constant introduction of the cocaine into the nasal area. These are very serious conditions and create a major problem. Of course, as mentioned above, the whole cocaine-cardiac phenomena is something to be kept in mind because one can develop acute myocardial infarction secondary to spasm of the coronary arteries, cutting the flow of oxygen to the myocardium leading to an acute MI and also cardiac arrhythmias. So sudden death associated with cocaine abuse does not always have to do with the fact that a person takes an overdose of cocaine (what will cause death also), but the very fact that one can develop arrhythmias and also acute myocardial infarction. There are a whole host of Myocardial diseases that are associated with cocaine abuse. That should really be used as a deterrent to deter people from getting involved in this

whole subculture of drug abuse. This material is toxic to many systems in the body and when one uses cocaine IV, the IV injection can also lead to hepatitis the same way it leads to hepatitis with Heroin because the needles are dirty and mixed with the bloods of other individuals who carry the hepatitis. And, of course the most devastating infection of all that can be transmitted with IV drug abuse is the HIV Type 1 virus.

INCIDENCE OF COCAINE USE

Again, it should be emphasized in terms of the cocaine situation, according to published data, more than 25 million people in the U.S. have tried cocaine. Some 10–15 million are regular users and anywhere from 5 to 7 million suffer from serious problems because of the use of cocaine. It is said that somewhere in the neighborhood of 5000–8000 Americans every day try cocaine for the first time. Again we know that cocaine is no longer a drug for the upper class. Many African-Americans find themselves involved with cocaine and crack cocaine.

To get help these individuals can refer to Cocaine Anonymous, 6125 Washington Blvd. Suite 202, Los Angeles, CA 90230. Tel. #1-213-559-5833.

OVERDOSE OF OPIOIDS AND OTHER NARCOTICS, AND THEIR TREATMENTS

The first thing (in the Emergency Room) is to establish the fact, "is the patient conscious?" If the patient is unconscious perform a neurological examination by looking at the pupils, while looking for focal signs (such as the Babinski sign). If the patient is unconscious, the patient has to be intubated so they can breathe, by providing oxygen treatment. At the same time of intubation, pass a gastric tube in to empty the stomach of the overdose substance. Also, use Ipecac syrup. If the patient is alert, then give the Ipecac which will induce vomiting within 30 minutes. Be very careful, because if the patient is semi-conscious and vomits, there is a possibility that, they, may aspirate the vomitus. This could lead to further pulmonary complication. If the patient is able to tolerate the material, then give the Ipecac so that they can vomit. If not, intubate them and then give them gastric lavage with normal saline. But one can't really try to gastric lavage in a combative patient because this could create problems.

At the same time that the patient is intubated and one is going to do a gastric lavage, it is important to put activated charcoal into the stomach. Activated charcoal should be given in the range of 500 to 1000 grams in 50–100 cc of Sorbitol. That is used as an absorbent to prevent more of the toxic substance from being absorbed.

Depending on the material that the person has overdosed on, it may be useful to use diuretics to get the patient to eliminate the substance through the kidneys. If it's a weak acid like aspirin use sodium bicarb and Lasix as a diuretic to eliminate the material. If the situation is more serious, resort to dialysis to try to remove the material.

If the person has overdosed on opioids such as Heroin or Morphine or Demerol, the antidote is Narcan. First give a prescribed dose of Narcan, and then set up a Narcan drip anywhere from 24–48–72 hours. A Narcan drip will eventually eliminate the opioids from the individual's body, check the vital signs, the pupils, and also check blood levels to determine if the opioid is being eliminated.

If the individual has taken an overdose of barbiturates, use sodium bicarb, diuresis, and activated charcoal to try to prevent further absorption. Again, depending on the level of consciousness, one may have to intubate the patient and do gastric lavage after placing the activated charcoal. If the patient has taken benzodiazipines, Ipecac syrup can be used to induce vomiting and also gastric lavage should be used with activated charcoal. But, if it's an overdose of cocaine don't do any of these procedures. Breathe for the patient, and provide oxygen for the patient.

Individuals who have cocaine intoxication will be combative, have confused speech, be anxious, and apprehensive. Also, they may have visual hallucinations, and they may feel things creeping on their skin. Also, they are very fatigued and irritable. If they develop cocaine withdrawal (about 24 hours later) they will feel fatigued, have insomnia, hypersomnia, psychomotor agitation. They may also develop cocaine delirium with violent and aggressive type of behavior.

Again, the most important procedure in dealing with cocaine overdose is to maintain the airway, control the cardiovascular system, and when agitation develops, resort to small doses of Valium or other benzodiazepines to try to control it. Sometimes, medication such as Haldol must be given to try to control the agitation and confused state. But anytime—from the time the patient becomes acutely intoxicated with cocaine up to 48 hours or so later—they can develop severe cardiac arrhythmias, acute myocardial infarction which can lead to death. Also, the long term use of cocaine and crack takes its toll on the brain with the possibility of the development of organic brain syndrome. There is also a 24 hour cocaine hot line, 1-800-COCAINE, that can provide information. There is also 1-800-262-2463 to try to help people who take cocaine, and are looking for help to get off of it.

As for those who want to get in touch with Narcotics Anonymous it is: Narcotics Anonymous, PO Box 9999, Van Nuys, CA 91409. Telephone # 1-818-878-3951. For those who are trying to get off of using marijuana, there is Marijuana Addicts Anonymous, PO Box 1969, Bowling Green Station, New York, NY 10274. Tel. # 1-212-459-4423.

AMPHETAMINE OVERDOSES AND THEIR TREATMENTS

Give them Ipecac syrup and diuresis and in this case acidify the urine, gastric lavage, activated charcoal, hemodialysis applies. If it is benzodiazipine, again give them Ipecac, gastric lavage, and activated charcoal. If its the hypnotics, Ipecac syrup will induce vomiting within 30 minutes. Gastric lavage is important plus activated charcoal. Phenothiazides use Ipecac syrup, gastric lavage and activated charcoal.

There are other drugs that these people can take an overdose of such as phencyclidine. Sometimes this condition can lead to rhabdomyolysis which can lead to severe precipitous renal failure. Hemodialysis applies. Aspirin overdoses is very serious. Not only can this cause bleeding but it can stop people from breathing. The key is to really alkalinize the urine to try to get rid of the substance with diuresis. Gastric lavage with activated charcoal in the stomach and sometime dialysis to get rid of the aspirin. The same applies for Tylenol type medications. Again gastric lavage, alkalinize the urine, give Lasix. There is also the substance that is used called Mucomist and another name for it is actylcysteine. This can be used to reverse the effect of the liver toxicity of Tylenol and it is basically given at 40 mg. per kilogram by mouth and then add 70 mg. per kilogram every 4 hours up to 17 doses. Too much Tylenol can kill someone and the toxicity of the liver begins anywhere from 48 to 100 hours. It's very important to know this and keep this medication going for up to 17 doses trying to reverse the effect of these conditions. Also if one overdoses on alcohol, it is going to depress respirations. Therefore, get control of the breathing mechanism by intubating the patient.

Amphetamine overdose is also associated with seizures. Again, the barbituates are respiratory depressants, so control of the respiratory system, providing appropriate oxygen, is extremely necessary.

HEROIN OVERDOSE AND ITS TREATMENT

With Heroin overdose, there is meiosis, pinpoint pupils, and there will be trouble breathing. Also, the mental status may be depressed. The antidote is anywhere from .4 to 2 mg. of Narcan, sometimes up to 10 mg. of Narcan. Narcan has a short life of about 60 minutes. Sometimes a Narcan drip must be kept going for, as stated above, anywhere from 24 to 72 hours.

The important thing to realize about these drugs, is that an overdose can actually kill. Something as mundane as aspirin can cause severe acidosis with central nervous system side effects. This can lead to severe bleeding associated with the GI tract. When one takes too much aspirin, gastritis leading to anemia which can also lead to shock and death. If this condition is not handled properly and because of the massive amount of blood that may be lost, it can be fatal.

The tricyclics medication can cause hypotension and drying of the mouth. A whole host of cardiac arrhythmias can occur because of an overdose of these medications. These are very dangerous medications, and if one takes an overdose, get prompt medical attention. If the hospital is not well equipped and the emergency room staff are not well versed on how to handle an overdose, then the patient is already doomed. Unfortunately, in the case of the African-Americans this occurs because they are not likely to get prompt care in the medical setting.

However, they are better off in a big teaching hospital where you are likely to have residents in training that are more up to date in terms of how to handle these problems as opposed to a tiny small community hospital where there is often only one doctor in the emergency room and he/she may not be able to handle the situation but that is the chance that one is taking. So if possible to rush these patients if they get picked up by an EMS to rush them to the biggest city hospital around in the area so that they can get the appropriate care they need to combat the overdoses of these very lethal substances which leads to a tremendous amount of death every year because of overdose of these substances.

If the patient did not aspirate and has no serious pulmonary or cardiac complications then the patient gets acute care. Also, he/she is kept NPO and receives IV fluids with either D5 normal saline or Ringer's lactate. Also, he/she should be kept under watch for possible seizure developments. Then, the patient should be seen by the psychiatrist to make sure that this was not an attempt at suicide. Next, the patient is advised in terms of long term treatment of abstinence for the substance the patient was abusing. The patient should get a complete blood count, liver chemistries, chest X-ray, EKG. Sometime, there may be an abnormal blood count associated with this acute problem. There may be an acute leukemoid reaction with a high white count, high platelet count. Or, there may be an acute situation whereby the white count is low because of acute marrow suppression that leads to a low white count, low red count, low platelet count and pancytopenia secondary to the acute toxicity of these drugs to the bone marrow. One may see this acutely and are dealing with the blood dyscrasias. If there are cardiac arrhythmias, treat appropriately by keeping the patient on the monitor. Sometimes, if they have pvc's they have to be treated with Lidocaine and sometimes procainamide depending on the type of arrhythmias they are having. They may have atrial fibrillation or paroxysmal atrial fibrillation and have to be treated with digitalis transiently, etc.

After it is documented that they are not having seizures, they may have to be given small doses of medications such as Ativan, Valium and Librium. Later, try to gradually taper them off their medications. To prevent them from going into withdrawal, give them small doses of Valium or Haldol while trying to gradually taper down.

Check the patient's overall health in terms of the different types of venereal diseases that these individuals bring with them into the hospital. A VDRL is done and frequently one finds that the male has a penile discharge, and have to be cultured, a gram stain has to be done and he has to be treated for gonorrhea and chlamydia and sometimes herpes. One may have to treat them for infectious diseases such as tuberculosis, in particular if one finds that the chest x-ray shows an abnormality such as an infiltrate that could be consistent with a diagnosis of tuberculosis. Place a PPD or tine test on the person's forearm, culture the sputum for TB and stain the sputum for AFB. If there is a strong suspicion of TB based on the AFB stain, then the patient must be treated with anti-TB medications, while waiting for the result of the TB culture from the lab, which usually takes six weeks. These patients also carry a high incidence of HIV, so when they come into the hospital they should have an HIV test done.

INFECTIONS ASSOCIATED WITH DRUG ADDICTION

It is not enough to just admit the patient for a drug problem. Associated with the drug problem is a high incidence of infectious diseases and sexually transmitted diseases. AIDS, herpes, syphilis, gonorrhea, chlamydia and all these common infections. Tuberculosis is also a common infection that affects these individuals.

In summary, drug addiction is a serious disease with life-long implications for the individual who is addicted. It has multi-system potential and severe psycho-social abnormalities associated with it. Once an addict, the individual must make a lifetime commitment to refrain from using addicting drugs through drug treatment programs. It is important not to take the first puff of an addicting drug, the first snort of an addicting drug, the first injection of an addicting drug and the first tablet of an addicting drug, unless prescribed by a physician for a specific disease-associated condition. The addicting nature of these substances are such that once you start, it is very hard to stop, so therefore, don't start using drugs—period, and if you are already using drugs now, seek immediate help from a drug treatment program.

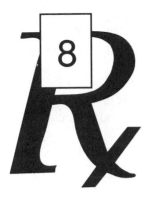

ANEMIA

CHAPTER OUTLINE

Definition of Anemia

Different Types of Anemia

Bone Marrow

Bone Marrow Failure

Definition of Alpha Thalassemia

Hypoproliferation of Bone Marrow

Iron Deficiency Anemia

Iron Deficiency in Men

Serum Ferritin

Different Types of Microcytic
Hypochromic Anemia

Red Cells Distribution Width (RDW)
in Iron Deficiency Anemia

Evaluation of Iron Deficiency
Anemia in Men

Treatment of Iron Deficiency Anemia

Vitamin C in Iron Deficiency Anemia

Signs and Symptoms of Iron Deficiency
Anemia

Incidence of Iron Deficiency Anemia

Poverty and Iron Deficiency Anemia

Alcohol Abuse and Iron Deficiency
Anemia

PICA and Iron Deficiency Anemia

Tea Drinking and Iron Deficiency Anemia

Aspirin and Its Effects on the Stomach

Non-Steroidal Anti-Inflammatory
Medications (Pills for Arthritis) and
Their Effects on the Stomach

Cytotec and Its Effects on the Stomach
to Prevent Bleeding

H2 Blockers and Their Effects on
the Stomach to Prevent GI Bleeding

Sickle Cell Anemia

DEFINITION OF ANEMIA

Different Types of Anemia

In order for an individual to become anemic, one of three events must occur. 1) either the individual is not generating enough red cells; 2) the individual is bleeding; 3) or the individual is hemolyzing, (breaking up the red cells).

Bleeding can occur as the result of an accident, surgery, menstrual blood loss, bleeding from the GI tract, the colon, or the stomach. Also, bleeding from chronic hematuria as a result of disease may lead to anemia. Also, the coughing up of blood as the result of certain conditions involving the lung, Goodpasture's syndrome or pulmonary hemosiderosis, may contribute to an anemic condition. The losing of blood through the urine due to bleeding from the bladder or the kidneys is another condition that may cause anemia.

BONE MARROW

Chronic loss of iron may also occur as a result of a condition called paroxysmal hemoglobinuria (PNH). Not generating enough red cells could be due to infiltration of the bone marrow with cancer, or infiltration of the bone marrow with a condition such as Gaucher's disease (abnormal fat storage that can infiltrate the bone marrow).

BONE MARROW FAILURE

Also, bone marrow can fail as in aplastic anemia, pure red cell aplasia, or suppression of the bone marrow by an acute viral infection. An acute bacterial infection can suppress the bone marrow. Chronic renal disease, chronic liver disease, rheumatoid arthritis and chronic inflammatory conditions such as dermatomyositis, systemic sclerosis (scleroderma) and lupus erythematosus (SLE) can cause anemia.

These types of diseases can lead to bone marrow hypoplasia, which leads to the inability to produce enough red cells. Conditions that can lead to breaking up of red cells are: drug induced hemolysis, auto-immune hemolysis, (breaking of red cells through walking distances), chronic hemolytic disease, (sickle cell disease), hereditary spherocytosis, the thalassemias, both beta-type thalassemias, and alpha-type thalassemias.

DEFINITION OF ALPHA THALASSEMIA

In alpha thalassemia, one starts to become anemic when two alpha chains are missing. When three alpha chains are missing, this condition is called hemoglobin H. When four alpha chains are missing, this is called hydrops fetalis, which is incompatible with life and causes death (in utero). Hemolytic disease associated with cold agglutinin diseases can also cause brisk hemolysis to occur. Hemolytic anemia is associated with the complication of blood transfusion and can also cause hemolysis to occur leading to anemia.

HYPOPROLIFERATION OF BONE MARROW

Hypoproliferation of the bone marrow due to some vitamin deficiencies such as B-12 deficiencies, folic acid deficiencies, other elemental deficiencies such as iron deficiency can lead to anemia.

IRON DEFICIENCY ANEMIA

Iron deficiency anemia is one of the commonest diseases in the world. According to the World Health Organization record, 30% of the world population suffers from iron deficiency anemia. This amounts to 1.3 billion people. Iron deficiency anemia is the number one disease that affects women the world over, and there is a higher incidence of iron deficiency anemia in Blacks than in their white counterpart. This is due to the fact that Blacks generally eat a diet that is poorer in iron content than their white counterparts. The requirement for iron in men and post menopausal women is 1 mg per day. Menstruating women, because they lose up to four times more iron than men, require up to four times more iron per day in order to replenish that which is lost during menstruation. Also, more iron is needed during infancy. The recommended dose is 1.5 mg per kg of body weight. During childhood, the recommended dose is up to 10 mg per day. In order for an individual to achieve the daily requirement of iron, one needs to eat 10–20 mg of iron in the diet per day.

As mentioned previously, the reason why iron deficiency anemia is so prevalent in women is because women lose iron via menstrual blood loss every month. Complications arise in the case of the African-American women and other minorities because they are generally eating a diet that is poor in iron content to begin with. Also, coupled with menstrual blood loss is a tendency toward multiple deliveries of children who require breast feeding. A significant percentage of minority women have a loss of iron during pregnancy. This iron is not replaced in the diet. Through the combination of these factors, it is easy to see why iron deficiency anemia in the African-American women and other minorities is so much higher than in their white counterpart.

As stated, in premenopausal women, the number one cause of iron deficiency anemia is menstrual blood loss and childbirth. In postmenopausal, it's a combination of previous blood loss secondary to childbirth resulting in an iron loss that was never replaced. This is coupled with the possibility of blood loss from GI bleeding. Hence, if a woman is 40 years old and she has iron deficiency anemia, it is very important to evaluate the woman's GI tract to be certain that the iron deficiency is not just the result of previous menstrual blood loss or blood loss due to child bearing. Also, it should be evaluated to make sure that it is not due to GI blood loss, (the incidence of colorectal cancer is higher in women than in men). Therefore, at age 40 or older, a woman who comes to the office with iron deficiency anemia ought to have an evaluation of the GI tract with a sigmoidoscopy, barium enema, or a colonoscopic exam. If these are normal, then an upper GI series and small bowel exam should follow. Also, one should look at the esophagus, stomach, and the small bowel to make certain that there is no malignancy or ulcers in the stomach to explain the blood loss.

IRON DEFICIENCY IN MEN

Iron deficiency anemia in men is almost always the result of GI blood loss. A few conditions associated with iron deficiency such as Goodpasture's disease, pulmonary hemosiderosis, or other iron blood loss associated with the kidneys are so very rare that it would be unwise to consider these conditions first. The first procedure to consider in a man who has iron deficiency anemia is a thorough evaluation of the GI tract to rule out the possibility of cancer. If this is ruled out, one should try to rule out the possibility of an ulcer in order to explain the blood loss.

Other conditions associated with iron deficiency anemia are parasitic infestation causing chronic bleeding that results in iron deficiency. Also, other conditions to be considered in an athlete is iron deficiency anemia resulting from blood loss associated with bleeding that is the result of jogging, or other strenuous exercises. These can lead to splanchnic ischemia that can lead to bleeding in the large bowel. This type of bleeding is often seen in both men and women who are involved in running as a form of exercise.

Another case of iron deficiency anemia is the situation where men or women have undergone gastrectomies secondary to ulcer of the stomach. This is because a significant surface of iron absorbing area, namely the duodenum, has been removed. Because of this, the possibility of iron deficiency anemia in the immediate future has to be considered because of the malabsorption of iron. One must note that iron is absorbed mostly in the duodenum. Anytime there is any type of malabsorption regardless of the underlying cause, it can lead to deficiency anemia.

The total iron found in the body of a man is 3.5 grams; the total found in the body of women is 2.5 grams. The total number of iron in the man's store is 1.5 grams, and in the women it is about 1 gram. The best way to measure this is through serum ferritin.

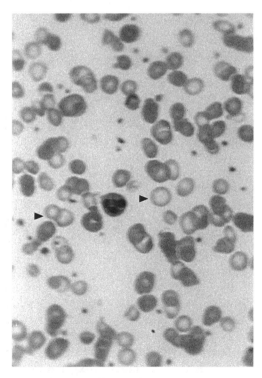

Figure 8.1. Iron Deficiency Anemia. Peripherial blood smear showing hypochromic pale red cell showing lack of hemoglobin. (arrow head) Arrow showing microcytic red cell (small red cell) due to lack of hemoglobin.

SERUM FERRITIN

The serum ferritin is a very easy test that can be performed in a doctor's office. It is a very effective evaluation of the total body iron store. But, there is a problem, however, with testing the serum ferritin because it is a phase reacting protein. Because of inflammation, infection, or cancer, one can have a falsely elevated serum ferritin. It is very important to keep this in mind. Serum iron and Total Iron Binding Capacity (TIBC) can be very misleading. The best test to evaluate the iron store is really bone marrow testing and staining of the iron. However, this is an invasive procedure and it can cause discomfort.

Women are expected to have a serum ferritin up to 126 N.G. If it happens to be 40, then it is low. This means that she is losing her store of iron in some fashion. The first iron to be lost when a person is bleeding chronically and slowly is the iron in store. This condition precedes iron deficiency anemia by several steps and several months.

The decreased iron store is called iron deficiency erythropoiesis (decreased iron storage). At this point, the patient has already began to feel the effect of iron deficient erythropoiesis by feeling weak, irritable, and lacking the ability to concentrate. This is because all the iron in store has been depleted. The individual is now operating only with the iron in circulation. Once this iron is depleted, the appearance of microcytosis (small red cells) sets in. This is reflected by a low MCV (mean corpuscular volume) ultimately leading to an obvious microcytic hypochromic anemia.

DIFFERENT TYPES OF MICROCYTIC HYPOCHROMIC ANEMIA

Microcytic hypochromic anemia has a differential diagnosis of its own. It is important to understand that by the time one develops hypochromic microcytic anemia secondary to an iron deficiency state, this process of losing the store of iron in a stepwise fashion, has been going on for several months, sometimes as long as a year.

The next level is when one begins to exhaust the iron in the circulation. It takes from 6–8 months for this to happen depending on how fast the blood is being lost. If the blood is being lost slowly, this process also takes place slowly.

Microcytic hypochromic anemia is a differential diagnosis which includes iron deficiency anemia, thalassemia (both beta thalassemia major and minor) and alpha thalassemia which involves the loss of two or more alpha chains in the hemoglobin. This will have a low MCV with hypochromic microcytic indices. However, in the thalassemic syndrome almost always there is a high total red cell count. This should indicate that there is a thalassemic syndrome as opposed to the iron deficiency anemia.

RED CELLS DISTRIBUTION WIDTH (RDW) IN IRON DEFICIENCY ANEMIA

Another index that may be used to arrive at the possibility of iron deficiency anemia is the increase in the RDW (Red Cell Distribution Width). One has to be very careful with this index because macrocytosis and microcytosis will increase the RDW. Sometimes, if there is a combination of microcytosis and macrocytosis occurring at the same time, this can cancel out the RDW. It is conceivable that a person may be hemolyzing for a variety of reasons, such as an auto immune disease and at the same time have an underlying iron deficiency state. There may also be a situation where one cancels out the RDW, and the RDW appears to be normal. Because it can be confusing, it's always best to perform bone marrow aspiration and stain the bone marrow for iron. This will settle the issue of diagnosing if there is iron deficiency. At the same time, one may be evaluating for a

hemolytic process by discovering erythroid hyperplasia in the bone marrow. The best procedure to arrive at a diagnosis in this case, would be for one to perform a bone marrow as opposed to relying on serum laboratory tests.

In addition, sideroblastic anemia may also be present with hypochromic microcytic indices. However, there is a whole host of other conditions such as lead poisoning, treatment with isoniazid (INH), chronic inflammatory disease, neoplastic diseases, hemoglobin C, hemoglobin SC, hemoglobin S thalassemia, alpha thalassemia, beta thalassemia, all can cause hypochromic microcytic anemia. As mentioned, once iron deficiency anemia is discovered, one has to undertake an evaluation to determine the underlying cause. If it is in a woman between 30 to 35, it is reasonable to do a three day stool hemoccult test after a thorough medical examination. If this is normal, it is appropriate to treat with iron.

EVALUATION OF IRON DEFICIENCY ANEMIA IN MEN

On the other hand, in a man (regardless of the age), one has to undertake an evaluation of the GI tract unless it is obvious that the man is coughing up blood, passing blood from his urine, or has a history of chronic bleeding from the nose, etc. But, it would be dangerous to assume that it is coming from these conditions. It is always best to do a thorough GI evaluation or an evaluation of the large bowel with a colonoscopic exam or a barium enema. If this is normal then, an upper GI series with small bowel evaluation should be performed to try to determine why there is blood loss. There is always a reason to be found to explain iron deficiency anemia in a man. If the man comes from the tropics or is living in the countryside in the South, it's important to evaluate the stool for parasites. This is to make sure that there are no parasitic infestations that can cause a slow

GI blood loss which can lead to iron deficiency anemia. Once these procedures are determined and the source is found, (cancer, bleeding polyps, or an ulcer), then it has to be dealt with the appropriate iron therapy.

On the other hand, if the woman is 40 years old or older, then actually a GI workup has to be undertaken to determine whether or not there is an underlying GI pathology to explain the blood loss besides assuming that it is due to menstrual blood loss.

Once the cause is found, again one has to replace the iron via iron therapy.

TREATMENT OF
IRON DEFICIENCY ANEMIA

There are several iron preparations on the market. The best three are ferrous sulfate, (each tablet of which contains 60 mg. of elemental iron). Ferrous gluconate, (each tablet of which contains 37 mg. of elemental iron), and ferrous fumarate (each tablet contains 66 mg. of elemental iron). It is very important to understand that if one is taking ferrous sulfate, one ought to take 1 tablet (three times a day) because one needs to have at least 180–200 mg. elemental iron per day to be able to absorb a certain percentage (1/3 of it). If one is taking ferrous gluconate, one needs to have 4 tablets per day. If one is taking fumarate, 3 tablets per day needs to be taken. Other preparations that are available are not always reliable.

VITAMIN C IN
IRON DEFICIENCY ANEMIA

Iron is best absorbed when it is in the ferrous state, which is the Fe2 state. It is very important to realize that the iron is best absorbed when it is reduced. In the elderly where one may have atrophic gastritis, one needs to be supplied with small doses of Vitamin C to further reduce the iron and to enhance better absorption. However, Vitamin C is a reducing agent and it causes a neutralization of the hemoccult test that is performed to detect occult bleeding. So, if one is on Vitamin C, and the stool is tested for occult blood, it is likely to be negative. This could cause a dangerous situation. If one is passing blood in the occult fashion, an examination is undertaken by the physician, and the blood is not detected because of Vitamin C, that may cause cancer of the colon to be missed. Cancer of the stomach may be missed because one of the ways of determining these cancers is to examine the stool for blood. It is very important to realize that Vitamin C may be a very dangerous medication to take if not prescribed by a physician and prescribed for a specific reason. In addition, if vitamin C is taken in significant doses, (greater than 200–300mg.) it can cause mobilization of iron from the store into the heart muscle, the liver, and the pancreas. If a person had idiopathic hemochromatosis (which is reasonably common in the population, 0.005% people in this country have this condition); it is not a very good idea to take Vitamin C.

In addition, a large amount of Vitamin C may cause diarrhea, and can also cause kidney stone, etc. Taking vitamins in general is a dangerous proposition unless one can document being vitamin deficient.

Once one has been given iron therapy, one has to understand that the first iron to be replaced is the iron in the circulation. The first iron to be lost is the iron in store. After it is replaced, (in the man it is 2.5 grams in that range, women 1.5 grams of iron in the circulation), the rest goes into store in the form of ferritin.

SIGNS AND SYMPTOMS
OF IRON DEFICIENCY ANEMIA

The symptoms of iron deficiency anemia are irritability, lassitude and weakness. It is very prevalent in the world, and even more prevalent in the American population and even more so in the African-American population. The reason why it is particularly prevalent in the American population is because of poor diet. The food that is consumed does not contain enough iron. There is an epidemic of iron deficiency anemia in Black children because of the fact that they probably did not get the proper vitamins when the mother was pregnant, and probably they did not get proper nutrition after birth. Also, they are not getting the proper food as a child and, the food they do get is poor in quality and does not contain enough iron supplement to prevent them from the development of iron deficiency. Of course, without enough red blood cells being produced, one does not have enough oxygen to carry to the brain in order to function, think properly and achieve in school. So, if one is anemic, one is not able to concentrate properly and the chances of producing intellectually in school is that much less. This is another reason why it is so crucial that this problem be corrected. The nutritional status of the minority population must be improved. If the nutrition is improved, children will be able to achieve more in school and become more productive citizens, allowing them to make the necessary contribution to their family and society.

INCIDENCE OF
IRON DEFICIENCY ANEMIA

In summary then, iron deficiency anemia is an extremely serious disease. It is the number one disease in women the world over. 1.3 billion individuals suffer from iron deficiency according to the World Health Organization.

POVERTY AND
IRON DEFICIENCY ANEMIA

There is a high incidence of iron deficiency anemia among the Black population. This is because of the poor economic situation which leads to poor living conditions, resulting in an overall poor health status. This poor health status is the result of the in-

ability to maintain a diet that contains the appropriate amount of iron.

By way of correcting this problem, our society needs to provide the necessary funding to undertake better care for poor women that are pregnant so they get better prenatal care and nutrition, so that they can give birth to healthier children.

The wealthiest country in the world cannot afford to allow this large segment of its population to lack proper nutrition from something as plentiful as iron (that is so easily obtainable and reasonably inexpensive). Nutritious foods and education ought to be provided to poor expectant mothers. They should know that foods that contain iron include: chicken, fish, beef, liver, and milk and bread that is enriched with iron. Certain cereals are enriched with iron. These foods ought to be available so that they can eat better themselves and also feed their children better. When women are pregnant they ought to stay away from alcohol. Alcohol causes gastritis which causes bleeding which in turn causes iron deficiency. Pregnant or not pregnant, too much alcohol always leads to gastritis which is another process in which iron can be lost. Any irritation of the GI tract (from the effect of the alcohol) leads to blood loss in the GI tract.

ALCOHOL ABUSE AND
IRON DEFICIENCY ANEMIA

It is a fact that cirrhosis of the liver in women is associated with heavy menstrual blood loss. Once the liver is cirrhotic, it is not able to break down estrogen in sufficient amounts. This excess estrogen causes overstimulation of the uterus leading to vaginal bleeding which leads to iron deficiency. Alcohol will be discussed later. I will clearly show how damaging alcohol is, how it can cause anemia, both of an iron deficiency nature and also of a macrocytic nature.

PICA AND IRON DEFICIENCY ANEMIA

Another chronic habit that plagues African-American women causing iron deficiency anemia is a condition called PICA. PICA is an habitual ingestion of unusual substances, such as earth or clay, (geophagia), laundry starch, (amylophagia) or ice (pagophagia). Poor black women seem to be more prone to eating these substances when they are pregnant. This seems to be more prevalent in the South, West, and in New York City. But, poor women in every part of the world are afflicted with the PICA syndrome. Eating clay is the worst form of PICA because it tends to bind the iron in the stomach, preventing its absorption.

TEA DRINKING AND IRON DEFICIENCY ANEMIA

Iron deficiency anemia can become worse by drinking tea. In minorities and the poor, where the diet is so marginal in terms of vitamin and iron contents, drinking tea while eating food can lead to iron deficiency anemia. This occurs because tea has many acids in it, especially tannic acid. Tannic acid complexes with the iron in the stomach, preventing the iron from being absorbed. In a woman who is constantly losing blood menstrually and is either on a diet to maintain her weight or is eating a marginal diet because of poverty, drinking tea while eating a meal is really bleaching out the iron from the food.

The best way to drink tea is to drink it separate from the meal. Drink tea on an empty stomach because tea can bleach out the iron that is in the food.

ASPIRIN AND ITS EFFECTS ON THE STOMACH

Aspirin is a common medication which can be obtained without a prescription, it can also be a very dangerous medication. It is valuable in many instances. However, it can cause a lot of serious problems, chief among them being ulcers. The aspirin causes gastritis which can lead to ulcers. Anyone who is taking aspirin for prolonged periods of time, (such as individuals who have rheumatoid arthritis and who are forced to take salicylates) are likely to develop ulcers. The bleeding that aspirin causes in a chronic way leads to iron deficiency anemia because of the blood loss. Coated aspirin decreases stomach irritability; however, even then it is not 100% protective.

NON-STEROIDAL ANTI-INFLAMMATORY MEDICATIONS (PILLS FOR ARTHRITIS) AND THEIR EFFECTS ON THE STOMACH

All the non-steroidal anti-inflammatory medications, (pills for arthritis), that are sold over the counter and/or prescribed, have the propensity of causing irritability, gastritis, and bleeding from the stomach—leading to anemia as the result of blood loss. It is very important to realize that individuals who have osteoarthritis, rheumatoid arthritis, and other types of arthritic conditions that require medication (because of the inflammatory process and the pain that is associated with this disease) are at high risk for iron deficiency anemia because of recurrent GI blood loss.

Protective measures that can be taken are: don't take aspirin if it is not absolutely necessary, don't take other medications unnecessarily, and only take them when they are prescribed. If aspirin-type medication must be taken, take it along with Maalox, Mylanta or any antacids.

CYTOTEC AND ITS EFFECTS ON THE STOMACH TO PREVENT BLEEDING

There is a medication on the market called Cytotec. This medication is approved by the Federal Drug Administration (FDA) for the purposes of preventing ulcer production of the stomach from aspirin and non-steroidal anti-inflammatory medications that are commonly used for the treatment of arthritis and other inflammatory joint and muscular diseases. Cytotec is a prostaglandin analogue. It is quite expensive but it is extremely effective in preventing ulceration of the stomach when used in conjunction with the above-mentioned medications. The mechanisms of actions through which it prevents the development of ulcers are:

1. It increases local blood flow to the lining of the stomach.
2. It increases the level of bicarbonate thereby increasing the PH of the stomach.
3. It increases the production of mucus which protects the lining of the stomach against irritability of aspirin-like medications.

The usual dose is 1–200 micrograms every six hours. It can cause mild diarrhea and softening of the stool. It should not be taken by women who are of child bearing age in the first trimester of pregnancy because it can cause spontaneous abortion.

H2 BLOCKERS AND THEIR EFFECTS ON THE STOMACH TO PREVENT GI BLEEDING

Other medications such as the H2 blockers, (Zantac), Pepcid (Acid and Tagamet), can be used also to decrease the irritability to the stomach wall that leads to bleeding and iron deficiency anemia. Also, Alka-seltzer contains aspirin and when one is taking Alka-seltzer on a frequent basis, this can lead to bleeding from the stomach. This leads to acute blood loss anemia and it also can lead to iron deficiency anemia.

SICKLE CELL ANEMIA

Sickle cell anemia is a disease that causes severe morbidity and mortality in the African-American population; it is one of the most serious diseases that afflicts this subgroup.

The incidence of the sickle cell trait in the African-American population is 7.8%. There is about a 1/164 chance that two carriers in the African-American population will marry. If this marriage takes place, there is a 1/4 chance that sickle cell anemia will develop in the children. If this is true, there is a 1/650 chance that any member of this population will develop the sickle cell disease.

The rate for hemoglobin C in the African-American population is 2.3% So, if the African-American population carries the hemoglobin S chain, then the probability of someone carrying hemoglobin C and someone carrying hemoglobin S trait to mate and have children is 1/280. 1/1020 will have inherited the Hgb. sickle cell C disease. In the American population the incidence of beta thalassemia is .8%. Therefore, 1/3200 births would inherit the beta thalassemia gene which is also a severe form of thalassemia (William "Textbook of Hematology" 4th edition).

Sickle cell disease probably originated several centuries ago in West Africa. The incidence of the gene in the new world probably came from West Africa.

The first description of sickle cell disease in America was the result of work done by Dr. James B. Herrick, (a physician in Chicago), who in 1910 made this discovery in a 20 year old patient (a young dental student) from Grenada, West Indies. Later, the basic molecular biological defect that causes sickle cell anemia was described by Dr. L. Pauling in 1949. It was discovered that the substitution of Valine for glutamic acid at position 6 of the beta chain of the hemoglobin is where the abnormality occurs. This leads to polymerization and abnormal shape of the red cell giving it a half-moon shape instead of a disc like shape.

There are several different abnormal hemoglobins that cause sickle cell anemia, such as hemoglobin D, hemoglobin SC, hemoglobin S thalassemia, hemoglobin E. However, hemoglobin S is the abnormality that presents the problems of sickle cell disease involved in Blacks.

Sickle cell disease has a reasonably wide distribution from different parts of Africa, United States, West Indies, South America, certain parts of India, Saudi Arabia, Greece, Italy, Sicily, and Naples.

If two individuals with hemoglobin S trait mate and have children, there is a 25% chance (1/4) that their children will have sickle cell disease. There is a 50% chance that one of the children will have sickle cell trait. And, only a 25% chance that one child will be normal.

It is important to note that sickle cell disease is a very serious and complex disease. It causes severe emotional and medical problems for the person who is afflicted with it. It is a multisystem disease. Red cells carry oxygen to all parts of the human anatomy and since the sickle cell is not able to do so effectively, oxygen delivery to vital organs is impaired leading to serious abnormalities in these different organ systems.

The red cells become very sticky and lose their ability to pass through small vessels, and the cells become hardened and malformed. The cells have a half moon shape to them, therefore they are not able to pass through small vessels easily. This causes vascular occlusion, (plugging the vessels so the blood cannot go through). Wherever blood cannot pass, there becomes a starvation for oxygen in that area. Any area of the body that doesn't receive oxygen in the right amount, dies. Hence, the reason for strokes (at an early age) in people with sickle cell disease. Also heart attacks and myocardial fibrosis (secondary to

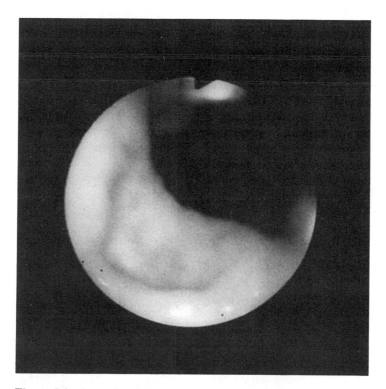

Figure 8.2. Arrow head showing bleeding gastric ulcer.

lack of oxygen going to the heart muscle) are caused by the disease. Also, there is a disease involving the liver, so-called sickle hepatopathy (abnormal liver). The spleen is also frequently destroyed in people with sickle cell disease because the spleen gets infarcted. Because the patient does not have a functioning spleen, it predisposes the individual to all sorts of different infections.

In particular, infection with bacteria that has a capsule is a problem because the spleen plays a major role in fighting bacterial infection. Disease involving the skin, and recurrent leg ulcers that will not heal are other results of sickle cell disease. Osteomyelitis infection (an infection of the bone) is often times caused by the organism salmonella as an indirect result. Children with sickle cell disease have a problem in growing because the endocrine system is affected in an adverse way, very early on. They cannot produce enough of the normal hormones that are needed for growth to take place. These individuals develop problems with the sexually productive organs. The children become underdeveloped because of their problems with sickle cell disease.

SICKLE CELL CRISES

In addition, there is a whole host of crises that occurs with sickle cell disease. For instance, the individual may have pains in the chest, the legs, and the abdomen, because of the lack of oxygen being carried to the tissue. The tissue is not receiving the needed oxygen so it develops anoxia.

Painful Crisis

Anoxia causes a secretion of kinin, which is similar to a blister bursting, which causes the tissue to burn. These individuals have painful crisis which lead to recurrent admissions to the hospital. Young people and those who are not so young slowly become addicted to Demerol and other drugs that ease the pain. It's almost impossible to have sickle cell disease for any length of time and not become addicted to these types of drugs.

Hemolytic Crisis

The next form of crisis is the hemolytic crisis. For a variety of reasons these people hemolyze more than the usual. They present themselves to the emergency room with a very low hemoglobin and very low hematocrit (because of the hemolytic crisis). A third form of crisis is the hypoplastic crisis. The bone marrow doesn't function properly, usually due to a viral type infection or any kind of bacterial infection. This is a very critical crisis, because without blood, and oxygen, one cannot survive. In a hypoplastic crisis, the bone marrow does not function, so the patient cannot function.

Hypoplastic Crisis

The way to determine if the patient has a hypoplastic crisis is to do a reticulocyte count. The reticulocyte count is the level of young red cells in the body. For a normal person, the reticulocyte count is anywhere from 1.5 to 2%. In a sickle cell person, they usually have a sickle cell count between 8–10%. If a sickler comes to the hospital with a reticulocyte count of less than 5%, then he's probably having a hypoplastic crisis.

Sequestration Crisis

Another form of crisis which occurs in infants is the "sequestration crisis." The infant develops a crisis whereby they suddenly go into shock. They have pooled the majority of their blood into the spleen, and there is no blood in the intravascular system. Suddenly, they have to be rushed to the hospital; if this condition is not recognized quickly and the appropriate replacement treatment given, they will just collapse and die.

The painful crisis is treated with IV fluids, normal saline, D5 normal saline or Ringer's lactate (whatever form of fluid is available). It has to be given in significant quantities, provided the patient does not have a cardiac condition, (as heart failure) that would prevent them from receiving fluids. After administering plenty of fluids, administer analgesics, such as Demerol or something even as strong as Morphine to try to control the pain. It takes several days of IV fluids and pain medication to control the painful crisis. Then, look for the reason for this painful crisis. Some people go into painful crisis because they are infected. It is always important to look for infection in a sickle cell patient because such a patient simply cannot tolerate infection. The polysegmented cells and the other white cells do not function very well. When they have an infarcted spleen, they cannot tolerate any infection very well. It's important to realize that the sickle cell patient probably has a white count of 13,000, and whenever one sees a white count that is above 15,000 in a patient with sickle cell disease, the patient is probably infected. Once the source of infection is found, the next appropriate procedure is culturing the patient. Look at the chest X-ray, and treat them with IV antibiotics. If the source of the infection is not found, look for the possibility of the hematocrit being too low. If this is the case, transfuse the patient. Transfusion is associated with a decreased incidence of painful crisis. It is important to transfuse the patient to maintain a good oxygen carrying capability so that the tissues can be perfused. This decreases the painful crisis.

The next step is the so-called hemolytic crisis. Hemolytic crisis again can be brought on by any type of infection. The patient is suddenly hemolyzing, and they have a hematocrit of 24–25%. Then, they have a hematocrit of 16–18. When they hemolyze, the reticulocyte count is likely to be very high. The patient then requires a blood transfusion. In addition to the transfusion, they need folic acid, which is to be given in high doses to patients with sickle cell and other chronic hemolytic diseases.

The folic acid requirement in a normal person is 50 micrograms. In someone who has a nutritional folate deficiency, one mg. is a mega dose. However, in a patient with chronic hemolytic disease (such as sickle cell disease), the recommended folic acid dose is up to 25 mg. per day. Most physicians don't seem to realize this so they keep treating the patient with 1 mg. which is not enough. It may be a mega dose for nutritional folate deficiency, but for someone with sickle cell disease 1 mg. is insufficient. This is because anyone who is hemolyzing is losing folic acid rapidly. One needs folic acid to generate new red cells in large amounts because one is also destroying red cells. So, therefore anyone who is hemolyzing probably has a definite folate deficiency. Therefore, 4 mg. of folic acid (four times a day) or 5 mg. (four times a day) is the recommended dose for someone with chronic hemolytic disease, (sickle cell disease). If they cannot take the folic acid by mouth because they are in too much pain, the folic acid can be given IV until the patient is able to eat.

So, in dealing with the hypoplastic crisis, maintain the patient with hydration, blood transfusion, and a high dose folic acid, until the virus abates. If it's a bacterial infection, after the appropriate cultures, chest X-ray etc., sputum cultures, urine and blood cultures, a broad spectrum is given. Broad spectrum antibiotics can cover both gram negative organisms and gram positive organisms until the appropriate culture results return.

As far as the sequestration crisis is concerned, there should be fluid replacement, blood replacement; folic acid treatment until the infant improves.

These are the four major forms of crisis that one sees in patients with sickle cell disease. And, sickle cell disease has a whole spectrum of problems that one has to be aware of.

Acute Chest Syndrome

The acute chest syndrome is a situation where the patient comes in with severe chest pain. They may have infiltrates in the chest that are not of a bacterial nature. They might throw pulmonary emboli (clots) and can develop adult respiratory distress syndrome. Some patients may even die from the so-called acute chest syndrome. Treat acute chest syndrome infiltrates with IV antibiotics.

GALLBLADDER DISEASE IN SICKLE CELL DISEASE

Also, the patients with sickle cell disease have a propensity to develop pigmented gallbladder stones. Most people in the population have cholesterol stones, but individuals with chronic hemolytic disease have, in addition, developed pigmented gallstones. And, it is very difficult for a patient with sickle cell disease to undergo gallbladder surgery because of the side effects of anesthesia and stresses of the operation. A significant percentage of these patients die as a result of their surgery. So, the patient has to be prepared appropriately, must be given hypertransfusion, have proper cardiac monitoring, must be given high dose folic acid, and be given oxygen therapy. Also, the hematocrit must be kept above 35% to 40% with hypertransfusion before operating on these individuals. If the patient comes in on an emergency basis with acute fever and septic like situation, it is best to bring the infection under control with IV antibiotics prior to doing surgery. Performing surgery on a sickle cell patient on an emergency basis increases the chances of the patient dying.

It is best to do gallbladder surgery or any type of surgery on a patient with sickle cell disease on an elective basis.

RECURRENT STROKES AND SICKLE CELL DISEASE

Recurrent strokes are a common problem. Children who are very young, in the pediatric age group ages 5, 6, 7 years old, have strokes secondary to sickle cell disease. The sickling phenomena is occurring within the brain, clogging the vessels and preventing oxygen from going to different areas. These children become ischemic and then an ischemic stroke develops. Again, hypertransfusion has some value in preventing this type of ischemic stroke. However, one has to keep in mind that the transfusion of blood has its own problems. Hepatitis B infection, non-A, non-B hepatitis infection, cytomegalovirus infection, and HIV type I infection (leading to AIDS) are to be considered. Because of the possibility of transmitting these infections to an individual who is being transfused so frequently, one must be careful and proficient. Physicians must give informed consent to patients for blood transfusions.

SICKLE CELL DISEASE AND RECURRENT INFECTIONS

People with sickle cell disease suffer from recurrent infections. In particular, recurrent pneumonias, most frequently pneumoccocol pneumonias because they have no spleen. Their spleen have been destroyed because of recurrent sickling within the spleen which causes infarctions leading to asplenia or hypo-splenia (meaning a non-functioning spleen). This results in a type of immuno-deficiency state resulting in frequent infarctions which are often life threatening. Infarction is the leading cause of death in patients afflicted with sickle cell disease. There is also an abnormality in the polynucleated leukocytes in the patient with sickle cell disease. These cells are incapable of killing bacteria compounding the sickle cell disease even more. It is important when someone who is a sickler and has an infection that it be detected quickly and appropriate antibiotic treatment is provided promptly.

BONE MARROW TRANSPLANTATION IN SICKLE CELL DISEASE

Bone marrow transplantation is being tried as a modality to try to decrease the transfusion requirements in people with sickle cell disease. There are studies on trying treatment with erythropoietin as a means to increase the hemoglobin F level and decrease the hemoglobin S level to prevent some of the complications of sickle cell disease.

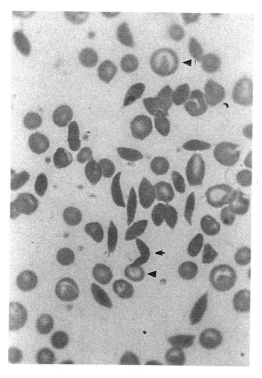

Figure 8.3. Arrow showing a sickle cell (banana shape looking cell) arrow head showing a target cell in a patient with sickle cell anemia with thalassemia combined (sickle thalassemia)

NEOCYTE TRANSFUSIONS IN SICKLE CELL DISEASE

In some settings there might even be the consideration of the possibility of so-called neocyte transfusions being done in patients with thalassemias syndrome and sickle cell disease.

HOW TO PREVENT THE DEVELOPMENT OF SICKLE CELL DISEASE

Family Counseling

Sickle Trait SA

If an individual has the sickle cell trait (the sickle cell S trait), then the individual has to be tested before having children with another person who may be a carrier. Remember, 7.8% of the African-American population carry the sickle cell trait. Therefore, counseling and testing should be performed to try to avoid having children with sickle cell trait from pairing and having a baby. Second, if somebody has beta thalassemia, avoid having children with someone with the sickle cell trait. If someone with the sickle SA trait has a baby with someone with the beta thalassemia trait, then there is 1/4 chance of developing sickle thalassemia.

Hemoglobin C Trait

This same rule applies to hemoglobin C. Hemoglobin C trait is found in around 2.8% of the African-American population.

HEMOGLOBIN SC DISEASE

If one has SC disease, avoid having children with someone with the S trait. One percent of the individuals will have the sickle cell C disease. Sickle cell C disease is just as serious as sickle cell S disease. As a matter of fact, sickle cell C disease is more devastating particularly to the eyes. Individuals with sickle cell C disease have more problems with their eyes that can lead to blindness than individuals with sickle cell S disease. Also, people with sickle cell C disease have crisis the same as sickle cell S disease. Everything as it relates to sickle cell S disease applies to individuals with sickle cell C disease.

MEDICAL COMPLICATIONS OF SA DISEASE

Individuals with sickle cell A trait also have problems. There are certain conditions in medicine that are associated with the sickle cell trait such as: splenic infarction at high altitudes, hematuria, recurrent bacteuria and pyelonephritis in pregnancy. Also, there is an association with pulmonary embolism, and renal papillary necrosis which occurs in people with sickle cell trait. Avascular necrosis of the bone (where the bone cannot receive any blood supply) is known to occur. Also, one may have actual sickling phenomena occurring after strenuous exercise. There is a condition called hyposthenuria (the inability to concentrate the urine), which occurs in patients with sickle cell trait. So, sickle cell trait individuals even though they have only about 40% of their cells sickling, may still have significant problems. Although they do not necessarily appear to be anemic and their hematocrit may be normal, they still will have certain problems because of the sickle trait cell.

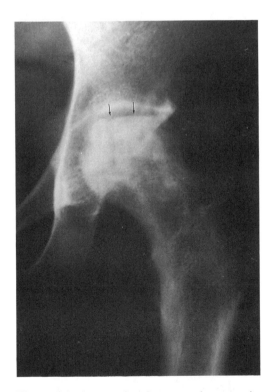

Figure 8.4. Arrows showing avascular necrosis (lack of blood flow to bone) of femoral head with flattening and necrosis of hip bone in a patient with sickle cell disease.

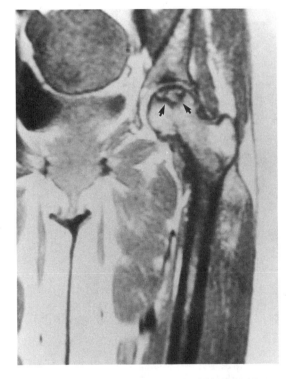

Figure 8.5. MRI of femoral head of hip of patient with sickle cell disease. Arrows showing avascular necrosis.

SICKLE CELL DISEASE
AND ALPHA THALASSEMIA

It is known that individuals who have sickle cell disease may carry the alpha thalassemia trait. When they do, there is a modification of the sickle phenomena. This is a positive situation in individuals who have the sickle cell trait because they usually have on their hemoglobin electrophoresis test 60% hemoglobin A and 40% hemoglobin S. However, if this individual happens to be carrying the alpha thalassemia and if they are missing just one alpha chain, they tend to have 35% hemoglobin S. If they are missing two alpha chains, the hemoglobin S decreases further to about 30%. It has also been documented that the individual who carries the alpha thalas-

semia trait and has sickle cell disease tends to have less severe crisis or they modify the disease to the point where there is evidence that they tend to even live longer. This is important because alpha thalassemia is indeed the most common genetic abnormality in African-Americans (about 32%). Only 2% of the African-American population is missing two alpha chains, (alpha thalassemia type 1) and 30% are missing one alpha chain (alpha thalassemia type 2). Therefore, there is a high incidence of alpha thalassemia type 2 in the African-American population.

Hemoglobin Constant Spring

It is, however, rare for a Black person to get sick from Alpha Thalassemia Type I

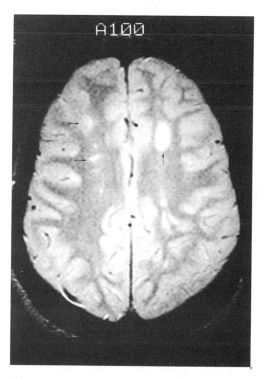

Figure 8.6. Arrows showing multiple infarcts (stroke) in the brain of a patient with sickle cell disease as documented by Brain MRI.

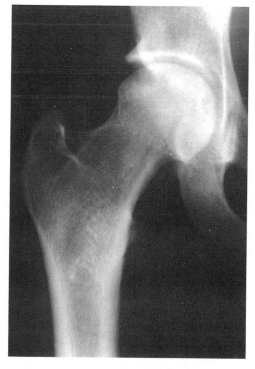

Figure 8.7. X-ray of a normal hip

because in Blacks, the missing Alpha Chains are located in the trans position—one Alpha Chain missing from two different chromosomes. In Asians, the two Alpha Chains are missing from the cis position on the same chromosome hence the reason why Asians who are missing two Alpha Chains get sick. This is called Hemoglobin Constant Spring.

As stated, sickle cell disease is a very serious but painful disease and the best way to prevent it is family counseling and hemoglobin electrophoresis testing. But just the screening test alone, (although it is an important test), it is not sufficient. This test only relates to the sickling phenomenon, but does not evaluate the type of disease or identify the sickle cell trait, or actually diagnose the sickle cell disease. The best way to diagnose sickle cell disease is to do a quantitative hemoglobin electrophoresis.

However, if one has sickle cell disease, one is likely to discover it very quickly. Infants with sickle cell disease start becoming sick from the time they are 1–2 years. But those with only the sickle cell trait do not always get sick. They may develop some complication of the sickle cell trait, but they don't get as sick as individuals with sickle cell S disease.

DIAGNOSING SICKLE CELL DISEASE IN THE FETUS IN UTERO

Now, however, the possibility of diagnosing sickle cell disease in utero has become a reality by examining amniotic fluid. By taking blood from the fetus any time after 6 weeks of pregnancy, a specimen can be taken (by amniocentesis) and the DNA can be evaluated. If the fetus is found to have sickle cell S disease, a decision can be made by the woman and the husband as to what option to follow. If it is SA, there's no problem to allow the pregnancy to continue. But, if it is an sickle cell S disease diagnosed in utero, the couple has an option whether to allow the pregnancy to continue and give birth to a child with sickle cell

S disease (with all its complicating factors) or terminate the pregnancy.

TREATING SICKLE CELL DISEASE PATIENTS WITH PROPHYLACTIC ANTIBIOTICS

It is also important to mention that individuals with sickle cell disease ought to be kept on prophylactic penicillin, (500 mg), Pen-VK (if they are not allergic to it) to be given every day to prevent infection from the pneumococcal infection (the commonest infection in this group of patients.)

If they are allergic to penicillin, they can take erythromycin (500 mgs.) every day as a prophylaxis. Also, there is a Pneumovax vaccine available that ought to be administered every 2 years. This is a vaccine against the pneumococcal infection which, as mentioned, is the commonest infection that these individuals become afflicted with. The Pneumovax vaccine is available to be given as an injection IM or subcutaneously (every 2 years). The pneumococcus is hardly ever found to be resistant to these antibiotics. Therefore, keeping the patients prophylaxed the year round is a very important clinical management technique to use. This is important to do because, as mentioned, these individuals have nonfunctioning spleens.

BETA THALASSEMIA

This is a disease that has a world wide distribution. It occurs in Greece, Italy, Asia, some parts of the Middle East, Saudi Arabia, Africa, Ireland, and to a smaller degree in African-Americans in the United States. Beta thalassemia differs a great deal from alpha thalassemia. Every normal individual has four beta thalassemic chains and four alpha thalassemic chains. In beta thalassemia, there may be a situation where there is a failure of production of the beta chain, either completely or partially. This failure may lead to the different types of beta thalassemias.

SERIOUS FORMS OF THALASSEMIA

There are several serious forms of thalassemia: thalassemia major (Cooley's anemia) and thalassemia minor, delta beta thalassemia, and persistent fetal hemoglobin.

Each different type of thalassemia leads to a different type of clinical manifestation. Thalassemia minor, which is heterozygous, usually does not lead to any serious problems, except in the case of stress brought on by example of a pregnancy, etc. Beta thalassemia has the ability to develop a complex situation when combined with sickle cell disease, resulting in sickle thalassemia. Anemia occurs in the beta thalassemias because of the failure of the beta chain, plus the accumulation of the alpha chain within the red cells. This causes precipitation of the alpha chain within the red cells, which causes precipitation of these alpha chains (called Heinz bodies). These cause early destruction of the red cells and further compounds the problem leading to severe anemia. Beta thalassemia hemolyses to a great extent—resulting in an iron overload. This is because the iron accumulates in the liver, the skin, the pancreas, and the heart. These individuals with this situation usually have bronze skin, and they develop a very large spleen. They also develop a failure to grow. They have abnormal looking bones with abnormal and deformed teeth. They die very early of cardiac complications

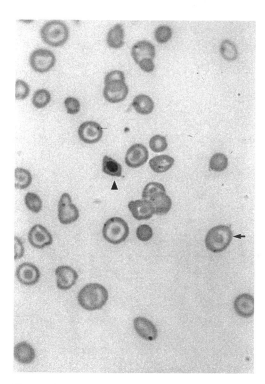

Figure 8.8. Thalassemia (arrow head) showing nucleated red cell small arrow showing Howel Jolly body. Big arrow target cell.

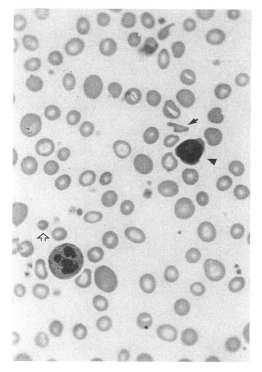

Figure 8.9. Hemolytic Anemia (arrow head) showing nucleated red cell. Arrow showing schistocyte (fragment of red blood cell) Open arrow showing spherocyte (very small red cell full with hemoglobin)

because of massive deposition of iron within the heart muscle.

Nowadays, there is the ability to diagnose beta thalassemia in utero using DNA techniques from the amniotic fluid. Also blood can be taken from the fetus using different techniques. If the appropriate DNA test is performed, it can determine whether the fetus is carrying this type of thalassemia or thalassemia minor. Therefore, a decision can be made by the expectant mother as to what to do with this pregnancy.

It's crucial to do genetic counseling to prevent the birth of children with thalassemia because of the suffering. As far as the African-Americans are concerned, again the same problem; lack of education, lack of exposure to the literature that needs to be discussed so that these individuals can take the protective contraceptive measures to prevent having these problems. Sickle cell disease, alpha thalassemia, beta thalassemia, sickle C disease, these types of conditions are all preventable conditions if the appropriate contraceptive measures are taken.

TREATMENT OF THALASSEMIA

Treatment that is available, in addition to blood transfusions and folic acid replacement, in this setting is a high dose of folic acid (20–25 mg. per day)[1]. Neocytes transfusions and treatment such as desferrioxamine subcutaneously using a special pump. But, most important of all is genetic counseling to prevent more beta thalassemic babies from being born to a life of suffering.

GLUCOSE 6-PHOSPHATE-DEHYDROGENASE DEFICIENCY

One of the most common abnormalities of red cells is a disease called glucose 6-phosphate-dehydrogenase deficiency (G6PD). This abnormality affects more than one hundred million people world wide. Those who have the full genetic dose of this disease have a condition called FAVISM when they eat FAVA beans. FAVISM is seen most frequently in Sardinia, Sicily, Greece and among Sephardic Jews. Interestingly, Blacks who are glucose 6-phosphate-dehydrogenase deficient are not susceptible to this condition. However, since 12% of American black males are glucose 6-phosphate-dehydrogenase deficient and carrying the A- variant of that abnormality, it is important to consider glucose 6-phosphate-dehydrogenase deficiency when a black male presents for medical care with an unexplained hemolytic anemia. This also applies to Greeks, Italians and Sephardic Jews; since all of them have a high incidence of glucose 6-phosphate-dehydrogenase deficiency among them.

Women from the sub-groups, namely Blacks, Greeks, Italians and Sephardic Jews can also be affected by this syndrome. However, with them the problem is somewhat different. The glucose 6-phosphate-dehydrogenase deficiency gene is carried on the x chromosome, therefore it is transmitted via the sex-linked mechanism. In men, only the x chromosome carries the glucose 6-phosphate-dehydrogenase deficiency gene and since men only have one x chromosome, men cannot transmit this disease to their sons because only the y chromosome is transmitted from a man to his son. In women however, there are two x chromosomes. One is affected by the glucose 6-phosphate-dehydrogenase deficiency gene, the other is not; so therefore, women who are glucose 6-phosphate-dehydrogenase deficient have two different populations of red blood cells in their circulation at all times. It is a matter of chance as to which population of red cells predominates. This will determine whether or not the woman will be affected by the factor that can cause hemolysis in a glucose 6-phosphate-dehydrogenase

[1]Source for high dose folic acid in chronic hemolytic anemia: *William Text Book of Hematology,* 3rd Edition,

deficient woman. If the glucose 6-phosphate-dehydrogenase deficient red cells predominate, then she is in the same situation as the glucose 6-phosphate-dehydrogenase deficient man and must therefore be handled the same way, medically speaking.

Routinely, this abnormality can be detected easily by drawing a tube of blood containing EDTA as an anticoagulant (to keep the blood liquid) and sent to the laboratory to evaluate for the level of this enzyme. A low percentage level equals a glucose 6-phosphate-dehydrogenase deficient state.

Before listing the circumstances and the different medications that can bring about hemolysis in this condition, it is important to mention that the glucose 6-phosphate-dehydrogenase deficiency gene is believed to have originated in West Africa.

The glucose 6-phosphate-dehydrogenase deficiency gene has meanings and implications in modern science that go far beyond it's disease-causing potential in these genetically predisposed individuals. Many of the hematological malignancies can have their genesis traced to the single original cell (stem cell) that brought about the full blown disease using glucose 6-phosphate-dehydrogenase deficiency assays of different types in the research laboratories. That is possible because glucose 6-phosphate-dehydrogenase deficiency is carried only on one x chromosome. By using different techniques, one can therefore trace the genesis of these different conditions plus many other interesting possibilities as it relates to the human organism.

There are different factors and different medications that can cause hemolysis to occur in glucose 6-phosphate-dehydrogenase deficient persons. Acute infections due to bacteria, fungi, viruses with high fever can bring about brisk hemolysis in a glucose 6-phosphate-dehydrogenase deficient person. Anti-malarial medications such as primaquine, chloroquine, dapsone, pamaquin; sulfur medications such as sulfanilamide, sulfaxazole, bac-

trim, gantrisin, sulfapyradine, nitr and other medications such as naladic and pyridium. Other medications that cause hemolysis in these individuals are: Isoniazid, Vitamin C, Aspirin and Phenacetin.

Anyone in the predisposed group of individuals above, Blacks included, who are traveling to malaria-infested places such as Africa and other parts of the Americas and the Caribbean where malaria may be prevalent, who by necessity, must be pre-treated with anti-malarial medications, such as chloroquine, must have their blood screened for the possibility of glucose 6-phosphate-dehydrogenase deficiency to prevent hemolysis as

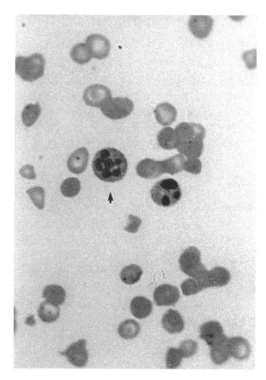

Figure 8.10. Folic Acid Deficiency in Alcoholism (Big arrow showing segmented showing polynucleated white cell with seven lobes typical of macrocytic anemia. Small arrow showing macrocyte (large immature red blood cell)

a result of exposure to these medications. The same applies to anyone with malaria who is about to be treated with anti-malarial medications. They must have their blood screened. The glucose 6-phosphate-dehydrogenase deficiency gene play a protective role in the malarial infested parts of the world (i.e. in Africa). Due to the fact that the glucose 6-phosphate-dehydrogenase deficiency red cells are not attacked by the malarial organisms, thereby sparing the individual the full brunt of the malarial infestation. In the large scheme of things over the centuries, this has helped to ensure the survival of these glucose 6-phosphate-dehydrogenase deficient Blacks who are living in these countries.

DIAGNOSING THALASSEMIC SYNDROME BY LOOKING AT THE BLOOD COUNT (CBC)

In iron deficiency anemia, there is an absence of iron stores in the bone marrow, low serum ferritin and also hypochromic microcytic indices. These conditions help support the diagnosis of iron deficiency anemia. On the other hand, in alpha thalassemia, there is a normal serum ferritin or elevated serum ferritin, and a more severe hypochromic microcytic indices, with a normal Hgb. A2 and normal Hgb. F. However, the RBC count per million is always increased in thalassemia usually, greater than 5 million with a low HCT and a low HGB.

On the other hand, beta thalassemia usually has an elevation of Hgb. A2 and also elevation of Hgb. F. Also, microcytosis is present which is more severe in iron deficiency anemia. The MCV is much lower than it is in iron deficiency anemia. Also, hypochromasia appears and target cells may be seen on the smear.

When this is coupled with an elevation of Hgb. A2 and Hgb. F, one has a description of beta thalassemia. However, it is important to mention that there is another form of beta thalassemia whereby there is a normal Hgb. A2 but the Hgb. F is elevated distinguishing from the above, whereby both Hgb. A2 and Hgb. F are elevated.

Presently, the treatment for this condition is the transfusion of the neocyte. Neocytes are young red cells, and by using special machinery, blood from a donor can be spun down. This sediments out the young red cells and they can be transfused to individuals with thalassemia. This allows the red cells to live a normal life span. Therefore, it does not result in depositing too much iron into the system. These individuals grow normally and have less complications of the thalassemia. However, this is not being done routinely. It is only being done in major medical centers, and it is rather expensive.

Individuals with these types of hemolytic diseases are also involved with the possibility of exposure to all sorts of infections because they have abnormally functioning spleens. In addition, frequent blood transfusions increases the possibility of hepatitis B, hepatitis non-A, non-B, CMV infection, and HIV Type A infection.

FOLIC ACID DEFICIENCY ANEMIA

Folic acid is a type of vitamin that is found commonly in bananas, lemons, and melons. Also it is found in liver, kidney, yeast, and mushrooms. The minimum daily requirement of folic acid is 50 micrograms. The maximum is 400 micrograms. The usual amount of folic acid that is found in the American diet is usually anywhere from 400–600 micrograms. In the total human body, the folic acid store is 5 mg. which is 5000 micrograms. So, if one's intake of folic acid is reduced to 5 micrograms a day, then in about 3–4 months the individual will become folate deficient. Folic acid deficiency is a serious anemia. It is usually seen in individuals who abuse alcohol to a great degree, or individuals who are on abnormal diets where they don't eat foods which contain folic acid. It's also seen in individuals who have malabsorption. This is because they are not able to absorb the folic acid due to some malabsorptive disease in the stomach.

Alcoholics become folate deficient because they don't eat foods that contain folic acid, and there are some reports that the alcohol itself can poison the folate pathway (resulting in folic acid deficiency). So, by definition, anyone who drinks alcohol excessively is likely to develop folate deficiency. Excessive alcohol intake is a minimum of about 60–80 grams of alcohol per day on a regular basis. Consuming the minimum of 60–80 grams of alcohol daily over 10 years is also likely to cause liver damage and damage to the pancreas.

The type of anemia that folic acid deficiency causes is called megaloblastic anemia. Megaloblastic means that the anemia causes the red cells to have an arrest in maturation. These cells don't have enough folic acid to proceed toward maturation and the red cells remain at the very early stage in the bone marrow. Therefore, there are not enough mature red cells in the circulation. Therefore, because of the arrest in maturation of the red cells, there is a lack of mature red cells in the circulation resulting in folic acid deficiency which develops into a very serious anemia.

The way one treats this type of anemia is first to evaluate the patient, and then one gets a blood specimen for the folic acid level. The red cell folate level is much more accurate than the serum folate level. However, the serum folate level is much more obtainable, and once one determines that the patient has folic acid deficiency, proceed to provide a folate replacement.

There is another condition that leads to folic acid deficiency. Anyone with a chronic hemolytic disease such as sickle cell anemia, thalassemia, hereditary spherocytosis or systemic lupus, and develops an hemolytic ane-mia secondary to it may become sick. Or, anyone who has the so-called autoimmune hemolytic anemia, because they are hemolyzing a lot of red cells, need more folic acid in order to replenish their red cell store, also need folate replacement.

FOLIC ACID TREATMENT

If someone is in need of folic acid replacement because of nutritional folate deficiency, then 1 mg of folic acid per day has to be administered. This is almost twice the amount that is needed for nutritional reasons. Usually a loading dose of 5 mg. should be given because they have been depleted for so long, and then a 1 mg. a day should be more than enough to replace nutritional folate deficiency. However, in individuals who have folic acid deficiency as a result of chronic hemolysis, they need much more folic acid than this. The recommended dose is up to 25 mg. per day. The reason for this large dose is because to generate cells destroyed chronically, one needs a large quantity of folic acid every day. Therefore, individuals with chronic hemolytic disease only, 1 mg. of folic acid is not enough. 20–25 mg. of folic acid per day is needed in order to correct the anemia, or at least to modify the anemia.

Individuals with sickle cell anemia and thalassemia are going to be anemic for the rest of their lives. However, they become more anemic if they develop a lack of folic acid.

So, folic acid deficiency is a serious condition, and it needs to be treated. Otherwise, there could be serious morbidity and/or mortality if it is allowed to continue in its worst form.

AFRO-AMERICANS WITH HEMOLYTIC DISEASE

With regard to the African-American population, since there is a significant incidence of chronic hemolytic disease such as sickle cell disease, it's important that these individuals be made aware that they need to take folic acid replacement. By taking folic acid replacement, they might reduce their need to have frequent blood transfusions.

Blood transfusion has never been a simple proposition. Now, it's much more dangerous because of the possibility of becoming infected with the HIV Type I virus leading to AIDS. Also, frequent and constant blood transfusions leads to a deposition of too much iron in the body which can lead to heart disease, liver disease, and pancreatic disease (result in type II diabetes mellitus). But, if one gives large doses of folic acid to individuals who have chronic hemolytic disease (such as the African-Americans who have sickle cell anemia), then the hematocrit is at a level in the low 30s, 31, 32% and the need for blood transfusions will decrease significantly. This is very important to remember. These individuals need large doses of folic acid (20–25 mg. per day).

B-12 DEFICIENCY ANEMIA

Vitamin B-12 is a very important vitamin. The body cannot function properly without the presence of B-12. Again, the total B-12 in the body of an adult is about 5 mg. The daily requirement for B-12 is up to 5 micrograms, which is a very small amount. The body loses about 0.1% of the total body pool of B-12 daily. This is 0.1% of the 5 mg. The foods which contain B-12 are basically meat, seafood, dairy products, and liver.

Since one needs so very little B-12 per day to survive (5 micrograms) and the total body is 5 mg., it takes anywhere from 5 to 9 years of total deprivation of B-12 for one to become B-12 deficient. However, B-12 deficiency is an extremely serious condition. There are many reasons why one can become B-12 deficient. One of them is, not taking any B-12 for too long a period or by staying completely away from food that has B-12. This is a rare event but it does occur.

Another problem is something called blind loop syndrome. Blind loop syndrome is when one has a blind loop in the GI tract (diverticulosis). The bacteria enters into a pouch of the bowel and remains there. There is a bacterial overgrowth and the bacteria literally eats away the B-12. In this particular setting, the folic acid would be very high and the B-12 would be very low (blind loop syndrome). Also, one could have B-12 deficiency because of sprue. Both tropical and non-tropical sprue occurs because of the lack of absorption of B-12 due to a malabsorption involving the GI tract.

There is also the so-called fish tapeworm. If one is infested with this tapeworm, the tapeworm will eat up the B-12 and the individual will develop B-12 deficiency.

PERNICIOUS ANEMIA

Another way of developing B-12 deficiency is a disease called pernicious anemia. Pernicious anemia causes B-12 deficiency because the body develops an antibody to itself and this destroys the intrinsic factor. The intrinsic factor is a factor that is needed to be able to hook onto the B-12 to help the B-12 to cross the barrier in the stomach and into the blood stream. So, when one has no intrinsic factor, one cannot absorb B-12. However, there is another condition that can lead to B-12 deficiency. If one has had surgery to the stomach (hemigastrectomy), and too much of the tissue that contains intrinsic factor was removed during surgery, anywhere from 5–10 years down the road, this individual may develop B-12 deficiency if the doctor is not prudent enough to realize the need for B-12 replacement therapy for life.

MACROCYTIC ANEMIA

The anemia that is associated with both B-12 deficiency and folic acid deficiency is macrocytic anemia. The way one diagnoses macrocytic anemia is when one receives the results from the hematology lab and this is placed in the Holter counter, one is going to see a large MCV (Mean Corpuscular Volume) of the red cells that are high (high MCV is macrocytic anemia). As stated, the two most common causes of macrocytic anemia are B-12 deficiency and folic acid deficiency. There are other conditions such as chemotherapy which destroys folate, DNA. Also one is likely to have a macrocytic indices. It is very easy to discover whether one has B-12 deficiency vs. folate deficiency. If one is anemic and the red cells count becomes too large, (high MCV), draw both folate levels and B-12 levels in the serum. Then, with these results, find out which

is lower. The standard by which to make the diagnosis is to perform a bone marrow aspirate to look at the red cells to find megaloblastic features. Megaloblastic features are associated with either B-12 or folate deficiency, whichever level is below normal between the folate and the B-12, that's the one responsible for the megaloblastic anemia.

When one is dealing with pernicious anemia, there is a whole host of other tests that need to be performed to make an accurate diagnosis. Because pernicious anemia is a very serious disease, the diagnosis must not be missed. If it is missed, then the patient is likely to develop serious problems that may have tremendous negative impacts. B-12 is absorbed in the terminal ileum of the small bowel. If one has disease involving the terminal ileum then naturally one will likely develop B-12 deficiency because of the inability to absorb B-12. If one had the terminal ileum removed surgically for one reason or another, the same thing will happen. One will slowly become unable to absorb B-12.

PERNICIOUS ANEMIA AND AMERICAN BLACKS

Pernicious anemia is a very serious disease that appears to have some hereditary predispositions. This is a disease that frequently affects the American blacks disproportionately as compared to other population. However, people of Northern European and Scandinavian extraction also have a predilection to developing this disease.

Usually, pernicious anemia is seen in people in middle age, but in African-Americans, it tends to develop at an early age, and it affects women, more frequently than men. It's a very serious disease because there is an autoimmune component to it. The body develops an antibody against itself, thereby destroying the intrinsic factor. Without the intrinsic factor, one cannot absorb Vitamin B-12. It is very important that

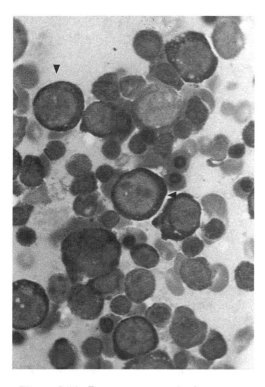

Figure 8.11. Bone marrow aspiration smear (arrow heads) showing megaloblastic red cells (very large immature red cell in pernicious anemia due to B-12 deficiency)

when an African-American woman feels weak and she is told she may be anemic, it is very crucial that she receives a thorough evaluation to make sure that she is not anemic as a result of pernicious anemia. Because, if she has B-12 deficiency anemia and it is not discovered early, there is a possibility that she might develop the so-called combined system disease. Individuals, who have B-12 deficiency, whether it is due to pernicious anemia or whether it is due to a variety of other reasons as mentioned above, can develop the so-called subacute combined system disease. This impairment of the neurological system results in a condition called spastic ataxia with degeneration of the dorsal columns. This can cause paralysis. Also the lack of B-12 can cause serious mental problems. Mental problems resulting in inability to think, concentrate, which may even lead to acute psychosis, and chronic psychiatric conditions. There are people in psychiatric institutions today, because (when they had B-12 deficiency) they were not diagnosed. And, by the time it was realized that they had B-12 deficiency, the damage to the brain was already permanent. So, B-12 deficiency is a very serious condition because of its associated neurological problems.

In addition, one has to understand that there is a percentage of individuals who have pernicious anemia who may, in fact, have cancer of the stomach. So, it is very important that one not only diagnoses B-12 deficiency, but also differentiates whether or not B-12 deficiency is because of other reasons, or due to pernicious anemia. If the patient has pernicious anemia, in addition to making the diagnosis (via the Schilling test) one also has to evaluate the GI tract to look for the possibility of underlying cancer of the GI tract that has a frequent association with this disease.

Other conditions that are associated with pernicious anemia are Grave's disease of the thyroid, hypothyroidism, and vitiligo. If the patient presents with megaloblastic anemia with a very low hematocrit, low hemoglobin, feeling weak, and has evidence on the complete blood count of macrocytosis, then one proceeds to obtain a B-12 level and a folate level. If the B-12 level returns low (the normal B-12 is between 200 to 900 ng) and the bone marrow shows megaloblastic changes, then one establishes a diagnosis of B-12 deficiency.

TREATMENT WITH B-12 BEFORE DOING SCHILLING TEST

To treat the patient with B-12, one must be very careful. One shouldn't try to do the Schilling test immediately because with B-12 deficiency there are megaloblastic changes. All growing cells in the body that require B-12 to grow are also megaloblastic which means, by definition, there are megaloblastic changes involving the lining of the stomach. If the Schilling test was given prior to treating the B-12 deficiency, there will be a false malabsorption pattern seen. So, one has to take several weeks to treat the patient with B-12 to correct the megaloblastic changes involving the GI tract before performing the Schilling test.

SCHILLING TEST

It is very important to do the Schilling test because one has to see if one is dealing with pernicious anemia or not. Also, there are blood tests that can be performed, such as, antibody tests to the intrinsic factor, or antiparietal cell antibodies, but in diagnosing pernicious anemia, the Schilling test results must be abnormal before one can be certain. The Schilling test is also important in that it can differentiate between mal-absorption and pernicious anemia.

Since 95% of people with pernicious anemia have antibodies against intrinsic factor and/or parietal cell, this blood test when positive, is sufficient proof that the individual has pernicious anemia, which makes the Schilling test unnecessary.

The way one does this is to inject the patient with 1 mg. of B-12 to saturate the site, and then give the patient B-12 tablets that have a nuclear substance in them (a tracer), to drink. After the patient drinks this, collect urine for 24 hours. Then, see how much of the B-12 that has the tracer in it has passed into the urine. This is only the first half of the test.

Repeat the test by giving the patient another B-12 pill with nuclear tracer marker, except at this time, provide the patient with an intrinsic factor. After the patient has taken both the B-12 and the intrinsic factor, the level of the B-12 that is excreted in the urine over the next 24 hour test should be in the normal range. Now, one has established the fact that the patient has pernicious anemia because by replacing the intrinsic factor at this time (which the patient is missing), there is normal B-12 in the urine.

MALABSORPTION

If both the first part, (the part without the intrinsic factor), is abnormal, and the part with the intrinsic factor is abnormal, one may make the diagnosis of malabsorption (which means that the patient cannot absorb B-12 either with or without intrinsic factor).

Again, if both parts of the test are abnormal, the diagnosis is malabsorption. If the first part is abnormal and the second part is normal, and one gives the intrinsic factor, one has pernicious anemia. After one has diagnosed the pernicious anemia, proceed to do an upper GI series to evaluate that there are no GI malignancies associated with it. Also, send tests for thyroid, and if the patient were to have vitiligo, it will clearly appear on the skin. Now one has to treat this patient for life with B-12 injections (once a month).

TREATING B-12 DEFICIENCY

The way one treats a patient with B-12 deficiency is to give 1 mg. of B-12 IM by injection intramuscularly every day (for 2 weeks). Then, give 1 mg. of B-12 (every week) until the hematocrit becomes normal. After this, give 1 mg. of B-12 (every month) for life.

Now, a word of caution is in order. If the person who has B-12 deficiency has underlying cardiac disease and is taking medication such as Lanoxin, diuretics, it is very important that one pays attention to what might happen to this patient. For instance, when one treats a patient who has B-12 deficiency, expect within 7 days to have an indication in the blood that there will be a brisk response to the B-12. Soon, the patient is going to start manufacturing tremendous amounts of red cells. The amount of red cells being manufactured, unless that patient had a problem to prevent him/her from manufacturing new red cells due to some chronic disease is tantamount to the transfusion into the patient of 2–4 units of blood.

If the patient has heart disease (such as congestive heart failure), and one did not take into account that this patient was going to have a brisk response, the patient is likely to go into acute congestive heart failure leading to pulmonary edema. This can cost the patient's life because of too much blood being manufactured, too fast, and one did not make provision to give the patient diuretics (such as Lasix) in preparation for the overloading of the cardiovascular system.

The second problem that exists is that in order for one to manufacture red cells, one needs to generate RNA. RNA is a substance that is needed for the production of new red cells. In the process of generating RNA one needs to use potassium. Potassium is a necessary substance for the body to function properly because hypokalemia, (low potassium), can cause tremendous muscle weakness and muscle cramps. It can even lead to the inability for one to contract one's chest muscles which could lead to respiratory arrest. It may also lead to lethal cardiac arrhythmias. So, it is very dangerous to give B-12 injections to someone with underlying cardiac disease without taking the necessary precautions. This is why it is dangerous for the patient to be asking for a shot of B-12. If the person does not need B-12 and they get an injection of it, nothing is going to happen to them because they didn't need it in the first place. They are just going to urinate the B-12 out. If, on the other hand, they happen to have been B-12 deficient and they get an injection of B-12, and they were not prepared properly for it, it can indeed lead to medical catastrophe which may lead to the death of the patient.

So, the person who is found to be B-12 deficient and severely anemic, and has been anemic for a very long time, frequently does not need blood transfusion. What they need is to be in the hospital and be worked up with a bone marrow, and B-12 level. Once the bone marrow and B-12 level is done, and one examines the bone marrow and finds it to be very megaloblastic (meaning that the young red cells are very large), one can give the patient some folic acid and B-12.

If the patient is elderly and they have cardiovascular disease and are anemic, they need more red cells to carry oxygen to the myocardium. They can be given a unit of packed cells very slowly with 40 mg. of Lasix I.V. Or, while they are receiving the blood, it is also proper to remove blood from the other arm which is usually very watery because it has very little red cells. So, they don't go into acute congestive heart failure by giving them this very viscous red cells. If you give this very viscous packed red cells to someone who has a hemoglobin of 5.5 or 5, they are likely to go into congestive failure. It is dangerous to be very aggressive by pumping a lot of red cells in someone who presents with a very low hemoglobin who has been anemic for a long time. If they are bleeding acutely, then they need to get transfusion of blood (2 units of blood), depending on the circumstances. But they have to get it very slowly, once a day. They may get another unit the next day, but each unit of blood should be given with potassium chloride replacement and then I.V. Lasix (or some other form of potent loop diuretic) so that they can urinate frequently while they are receiving the blood.

Another issue is the fact that the patient, as they are receiving B-12, is also going to deplete the potassium. Because they are using the potassium to make new red cells, they can become very hypokalemic and develop cardiac arrhythmias.

B-12 treatment is a very satisfying treatment because the patient responds so very well. But, it can also be a very lethal form of treatment if given incorrectly.

REMAINING ON B-12 FOR LIFE

After this is done, the patient has to remain on B-12 for life. This is 1 mg. of B-12 every month. The reason one gives 1 mg (which is 2 1/2 times what one needs) is because it's easier to draw up in the needle. If one just gives 1 mg. IM, the patient simply just urinates the rest of the B-12 that they do not need. The maximum B-12 that one can use on any one day is probably in the neighborhood of 400 micrograms.

B-12 DEFICIENCY AND THE ELDERLY

Another issue to keep in mind is that the elderly are very prone to develop B-12 deficiency (not pernicious anemia). This is because the elderly survive on a marginal diet that has very little B-12 in it. Another issue is the fact that the elderly have hypochloridia (the lack of sufficient acid in the stomach) because as one ages, one begins to produce much less acid because the cells lining the stomach also are aging and produce less acid. This leads to another condition called atrophic gastritis.

Atrophic gastritis is that when the cells in the stomach become atrophied for the lack of acid. And, without acid in a sufficient amount, one cannot absorb certain substances from the stomach very well; in particular such things like B-12.

Therefore, the elderly may present to the doctor confused with an inability to walk properly and all that may indeed be due to B-12 deficiency. The so-called "organic brain syndrome" is associated with old strokes and the whole aging process. This also may be associated with a lack of thyroid hormone as well as B-12 deficiency. So, when an elderly person becomes confused, the whole workup has to include a CAT scan of the brain to look for such things as normal pressure hydrocephalus which can cause these things, other significant pathology in the brain such as recurrent stroke or tumor. But, one also has to consider the possibility of hypothyroidism because there is a condition called apathetic hyperthyroidism which, in the elderly, can play havoc because the patient just simply withers away because of too much thyroid hormone production.

There is also hypothyroidism (a lack of thyroid hormone secretion) that can cause problems. Also type II diabetes mellitus with elevation of blood sugar with dehydration can cause this and, of course, hypoglycemia can also cause this. But B-12 deficiency is a very common condition that keeps people in a nursing home when they may not belong there. And, it also leads to a severe mental illness because B-12 is needed for the brain to function well. If B-12 is allowed to remain deficient for a long time, then anyone, regardless of age, will develop serious neurological problems, serious mental problems, and certainly serious overall medical problems. So, the whole syndrome of B-12 deficiency is not always associated with pernicious anemia.

EVALUATION OF THE ELDERLY PERSON AND B-12 DEFICIENCY

Therefore, then, in the evaluation of the elderly person B-12 deficiency ought to be considered. Just because it is known that B-12 deficiency can occur in the elderly, this is the very same group that it is wrong for them to be receiving B-12 empirically. Because, this is the very same group that are more likely to have a low potassium. Also, they are more likely to have congestive heart failure because of coronary artery disease. So, it is wrong for these individuals to receive B-12 without the appropriate evaluation.

FOLIC ACID AND B-12 DEFICIENCY

B-12 is an important component of the human anatomy, and it is a necessary component. If it is not present, then severe medical illness will develop as a result of the deficiency of B-12 in the body. Treating a patient who has megaloblastic anemia due to B12 deficiency with folic acid may partially correct the anemia while not correcting the B12 deficiency allowing for the progression of all the neurological problems associated with B12 deficiency. Physicians must avoid doing this.

CONCLUSION

African-Americans have to understand that pernicious anemia in this country affects more blacks than whites, and black females are affected more frequently than white females. Also, African-American females are affected more at an earlier age than whites. Although it is a treatable condition, it can lead to severe debilitating problems of a permanent characteristic if not diagnosed and treated early.

It also should be mentioned that there is a juvenile type of pernicious anemia that can be seen in the teen-age years if not earlier. The most important thing is that one ought not to start taking vitamins on one's own. When you feel weak, go to the nearest clinic, nearest emergency room, or nearest doctor so that one can be evaluated and have the appropriate tests performed. Nowadays, it is extremely easy to diagnose megaloblastic anemia because it takes 1 minute or less to put the blood through the Holter counter and the printed computer form will show megaloblastic features (an elevated mean corpuscular volume). If one knows how to interpret this correctly, this patient has a megaloblastic anemia and the possibility of folate deficiency vs. B-12 ought to be entertained right away. However, there are a whole list of other things that can cause megaloblastic anemia and an elevated MCV besides B-12 and folate. Suffice to say, people who are taking certain medications such as AZT for AIDS can have megaloblastic anemia. Individuals who are taking any type of cytotoxic agents for cancer, arthritis or other conditions for other autoimmune conditions where they are receiving cytotoxic agents, can present with megaloblastic features.

Individuals who are taking oral contraceptives can have high MCV because of a folate deficiency that is associated with oral contraceptive. These individuals who are taking Colchicine for gout can also have this problem. Individuals who are taking phenobarbital can have a high MCV because of folate deficiency associated with phenobarbital. People who are taking Dilantin for convulsions can have also folate deficiency because of the effect of Dilantin on the effect of the folate metabolism. It is also stated that individuals who are exposed to nitrous oxide can have B-12 deficiency. Nitrous oxide is a gas that is used in the dental field and when one is exposed to inhaling too much nitrous oxide, one can have megaloblastic anemia that can be very severe.

Megaloblastic anemia is easily diagnosed. However, anyone who is not a hematologist should not attempt to be treating B-12 deficiency or megaloblastic anemia. The hematologist ought to be consulted immediately once the suspicion arises that the individual has this condition. The hematologist is the best person equipped to handle not only the problem but the complications that may arise from this condition.

In order to take these precautions, minorities should actively take the opportunity to be exposed to the proper educational material that can alert them to these problems. Also, they should be tested to see if they carry this genetic problem so that they can try to eradicate the disease by not passing it down from generation to generation. Once they have the disease, they become dependent on the rest of society for the rest of their lives. They are not able to work although there are individuals with sickle cell disease who have managed to lead a productive life (but they are just a small minority). The vast majority of individuals with the sickling phenomenon are basically totally dependent on society, and it costs so much that there is no way a family can carry on by itself. These individuals almost always are on welfare and/or Medicaid so that they can obtain the medical care that they need. The key really is to try to prevent the disease by being informed about it and prevention implemented.

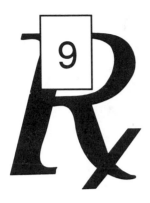

EYE DISEASE IN BLACKS

CHAPTER OUTLINE

Incidence of Eye Disease in Blacks

Different Types of Glaucoma

Cataracts

Diabetes in Blacks

Vitamin Deficiency and Eye Disease

Syphilis and Blindness

AIDS and Eye Disease

Reiter's Syndrome

Sarcoidosis

Sickle Cell Disease

Temporal Arteritis

Malignant Tumor and Eye Symptoms

Hypertensive Retinopathy

Hypertension and Its Eye Complications

Hemoglobinopathies and Eye Disease

Diabetic Retinopathy

Diabetes and Ischemic Eye Disease

Ophthalmologists and Optometrists

Syphilis and Eye Problems

Glaucoma and the Eye Disease

Open Angle Glaucoma

Low Tension Glaucoma

Secondary Glaucoma

Different Treatment Modalities in Glaucoma

Medications Used in the Treatment of Glaucoma

Cardiac Side Effects of Glaucoma Medications in the Elderly

INCIDENCE OF
EYE DISEASE IN BLACKS

Eye disease is a very common problem. According to the Center for Health Statistics in Bethesda, Maryland, 1.2 persons out of every one hundred individuals have some form of eye disease. Even though this is a high percentage overall, the incidence is even higher in the African-American population. This is because hypertension is so high among blacks which can cause a hemorrhage in the eyes which can lead to blindness. However, the number one cause of blindness in African-Americans is glaucoma. According to the American Academy of Ophthalmology, some two million Americans have glaucoma. Of that number, a very large percentage are African-American. For reasons that are not really very clear, and have yet to be found, glaucoma is more prevalent in Blacks.

DIFFERENT TYPES OF GLAUCOMA

There are basically four different types of glaucoma: 1) primary open angle glaucoma, 2) secondary glaucoma, 3) primary closure glaucoma, 4) congenital glaucoma. One fourth of all cases of glaucoma are present at birth and are due to congenital reasons.

CATARACTS

Another common disease of the eye is cataracts. The commonest form of cataracts is age related cataract, or senile cataract. Cataracts are basically an opafication of the lens of the eyes. The second form of cataracts is congenital cataracts, which is usually the result of maternal rubella during the first trimester of pregnancy. Also, there is traumatic cataracts because of foreign body injury to the lens or trauma to the eyeball. Also, there may be cataracts secondary to intraocular disease. Some cataracts are associated with systematic disease, such as Diabetes Mellitus, Down's Syndrome, hypoparathyroidism, and myotonic dystrophy. Finally, there is toxic cataracts, which are really the result of ingestion of drugs such as Dinitrophenol. This drug was used during the Thirties for suppression of appetite. The incidence of traumatic cataracts is higher among Blacks in particular, usually due to work-related circumstances.

DIABETES IN BLACKS

Diabetes is ravaging the black community, and as a result of this, the incidence of eye disease is also higher. Cataracts occur in juvenile diabetes also. One out of every fourteen African-Americans is likely to develop diabetes. This rate is 30 to 40% higher than that of other populations.

VITAMIN DEFICIENCY
AND EYE DISEASE

Also, nutrition must improve for African-Americans, because vitamin deficiency can lead to eye disease, Vitamin B-1, (Thiamine), and its deficiency can cause Beri Beri. There is an association with this problem involving eye abnormality which is associated with ocular motor palsy. This may lead to Warneke's syndrome, which is associated with ptosis, nystagmus and other types of eye problems. Vitamin B-2 deficiency can also cause eye problems. Although it is somewhat rare, there can definitely be neuritis associated with B-2 deficiency.

SYPHILIS AND BLINDNESS

Syphilis, when transmitted at birth, can cause blindness in infants. Herpes genitalis infection can cause problems with the eye. Other infections, such as toxoplasmosis, can cause congenital toxoplasmosis. All of these are associated with eye problems. As just mentioned above, infections can cause problems with the eye, viral, fungal or bacterial.

AIDS AND EYE DISEASE

Aids is an example of a viral infection that frequently affects the eyes. The eye disease that one frequently sees in patients with AIDS is retinitis. This form of rhinitis is caused by cytomegalovirus (CMV). Because the incidence of AIDS is so high in the African-American population, specifically about 29% of all AIDS cases in the United States is seen in African-Americans, AIDS associated eye disease is, therefore, quite high in Blacks in this country. (See chapter 10 for a more thorough discussion on AIDS.) There is no effective treatment for cytomegalovirus retinitis as seen in the AIDS patients. The two medications that have some efficacy are Zidovudine (AZT) and Ganciclovir. When these medications fail to work, the result is blindness.

REITER'S SYNDROME

Other conditions that can cause eye disease include Reiter's syndrome. Reiter's syndrome is a combination of uveitis, conjunctivitis and arthritis. It is very common to see this eye disease in drug addicts because they have a high incidence of venereal diseases such as syphilis, gonorrhea and nongonococcal urethritis. Also, autoimmune disease such as Sjorgren's syndrome may cause eye problems. Rheumatoid arthritis also has some association with eye problems, and all these diseases are seen frequently in Blacks.

SARCOIDOSIS

There is a high incidence of sarcoidosis in Blacks. Sarcoidosis often times presents itself with uveitis, which is an inflammatory process involving the eye, and can be the first sign of sarcoidosis.

Blindness can occur in untreated sarcoidosis of the eye. Black women particularly seem to be afflicted with sarcoidosis and its associated problems.

SICKLE CELL DISEASE

Another condition that has a predilection for the African-American population is Sickle Cell disease, both SC disease and SS disease. SC disease affects the eyes more than SS disease leading to vitrous hemorrhage which may result in blindness. If not treated properly with laser treatments, and even then, despite the best efforts, these individuals usually wind up losing their vision or having very poor vision. Individuals with Sickle Cell disease ought to see an ophthalmologist frequently.

TEMPORAL ARTERITIS

Another condition in the middle-aged to elderly individuals is giant cell arteritis, or so called temporal arteritis. This is a diagnosis that cannot be missed. Usually, the patient comes in with headache and with a general feeling of fatigue with some visual abnormality. The method to diagnose this quickly is to do an Erythrocyte Sedimentation Rate (SED rate). If the Erythrocyte Sedimentation Rate is very high, then the patient ought to be admitted to the hospital immediately, examined by an ophthalmologist, and started on steroid. Temporal artery biopsy should be performed as soon as possible, to support the diagnosis. If not handled properly and quickly, this condition can lead to blindness. A negative temporal artery biopsy, does not rule out temporal arteritis because this is often times a segmental process and a normal segment of artery could have been biopsied.

MALIGNANT TUMOR AND EYE SYMPTOMS

Another disease that affects the eyes is a malignant tumor, such as a primary malignant tumor of the lid of the eye (associated with xeroderma pigmentosum). There is also sarcoma of the eyes and malignant melanoma involving the eyes. Malignant melanoma is a particularly troublesome disease that can lead to the demise of the patient, so it has to be diagnosed very quickly. The eyes can also be affected by metastatic disease. Sometimes, eye symptoms are the first symptom of cancer somewhere else in the body. This is believed to be due to an autoimmune phenomenon (the body reacting to the cancer as a foreign agent, thereby producing an antibody against it).

HYPERTENSIVE RETINOPATHY

HYPERTENSION AND ITS EYE COMPLICATIONS

Hypertension, if left untreated, will affect many organs. Prominent amongst them are the eyes. The increase in pressure within the eye causes a variety of different vascular abnormalities. Since the eye is the only organ within which one can see a vessel, using an ophthalmoscope, it is rather easy to see the abnormalities.

Hypertensive Retinopathy is graded as 1, 2, 3, & 4, depending on the severity of the vascular abnormalities.

Grade 1 shows arteriolar narrowing.

Grade 2 shows arterio-venous nicking, some exudate and hemorrhages.

Grade 3 shows retinal adena, hemorrhages, and cotton wool spots.

Grade 4 shows a combination of Grade 3 plus papilledema.

If appropriate treatments are not provided for these abnormalities, the patient often develops blindness. Hypertension is a common disease, the latest estimate is that 62,000,000 people suffer from it, and close to 43% of that total goes untreated. This percentage of untreated hypertension is significantly higher in Blacks, since blacks most often are forced to do without adequate health care. Therefore, it is not difficult to see why there is such a high incidence of glaucoma and other hypertensive associated eye lesions, leading to a high incidence of blindness in Blacks.

HEMOGLOBINOPATHIES AND EYE DISEASE

There are different types of Sickle Cell Retinopathies.

1. Sickle Cell Disease Retinopathy (SS)
2. Sickle Cell C Retinopathy (SC)
3. Sickle Thalassemia

The most severe retinopathy between these three conditions is seen in SC disease. There are two types of retinopathies seen in sickle disease, the proliferative type and the non-proliferative type. The proliferative type

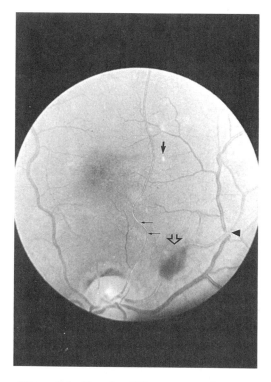

Figure 9.1. Showing different types of abnormalities in the eye of a hypertensive patient (hypertensive retinopathy)

Small arrow showing silver wiring

Big arrow showing hard yellow exudates

Open arrow head showing blot hemorrhage

Arrow head showing A-V nicking

is more common in SC disease and Sickle Thalassemia than in SS disease. These problems are due to sludging of red blood cells within the small vessel of the eyes. (The fact that the sickle cell is malshaped and sticky makes it difficult for it to pass through the small vessel). This then leads to occlusion of these vessels, resulting in a multitude of vascular abnormalities within the eyes. The types of vascular abnormalities seen ranges from arterio-venous anastomoses, neovascularization, resulting in leakage of blood from these new vessels causing different degrees of hemorrhages. Retinal tear and detachment commonly occur.

Fluorescin angiography is used to demonstrate these abnormalities. Photo-coagulation can be used as a treatment modality, and also laser treatment is used to treat these conditions.

DIABETIC RETINOPATHY

This is a devastating disease that causes blindness in a significant number of Blacks and other minorities who are diabetics. Some of the lesions that can be seen in Diabetes Mellitus are:

1. Micro aneurism
2. Arteriolar narrowing

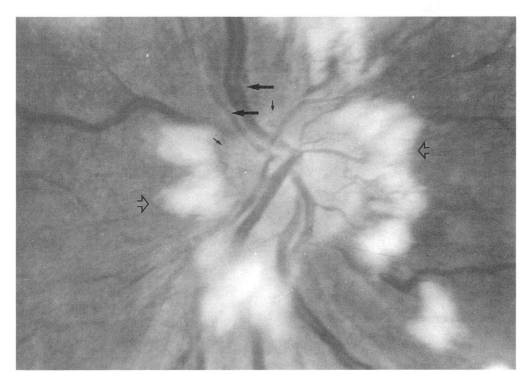

Figure 9.2. Showing different types of abnormalities in the eye of a hypertensive patient (hypertensive retinopathy)

Small arrows showing early papilledema

One big arrow pointing to vein engorgement (larger vessel)

The other big arrow pointing to arterial attenuation (smaller vessel); open arrow heads showing cotton wool exudates.

3. Retinal edema
4. Hard exudates
5. Venous abnormalities
6. Soft exudates
7. Cotton wool spots
8. Vitrous hemorrhages
9. Retinal hemorrhages
10. Retinal detachment

It should be noted that eye abnormalities may be the first symptom of diabetes. If the ophthalmologist is very astute and suspects such, he should recommend that a blood sugar test be done. If the diabetic retinopathy is not very advanced, the fact that the blood sugar is very high is enough to cause eye symptoms, like blurry vision.

Once the patient presents with symptoms of diabetes and is diagnosed with diabetes, the internist, the pediatrician, the endocrinologist should work closely in conjunction with the ophthalmologist so that

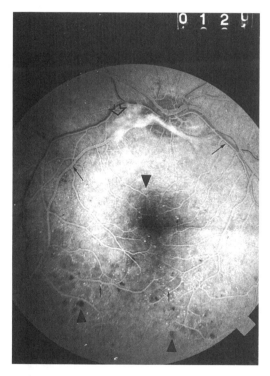

Figure 9.3. Showing different degrees of abnormalities in the eye of a patient with diabetes mellitus (diabetic retinopathy)

Fluorescein angiogram shortly after injection of dye in patient eye

Dye in arteries (white) and just starting to enter veins (large arrow)

White area off NH is neovascular tuff (open arrow

Black spots are hemorrhages (arrow heads)

Tiny white dots are microaneurisms (small arrow)

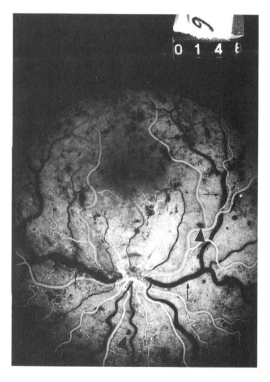

Figure 9.4. Showing different degrees of abnormalities in the eye of a patient with diabetes mellitus (diabetic retinopathy)

Large arrows showing dilated veins

Arrow heads showing hemorrhages inside the eye

appropriate care can be given to prevent unnecessary blindness due to diabetes. Because the incidence of diabetes is on the rise both in the African-American community and the Hispanic community, blindness is also on the rise because of its association with diabetic retinopathy. It is very, very important that the Blacks understand that if they present themselves to the doctor early enough and remain under constant care of a qualified ophthalmologist, they can prevent eventual blindness secondary to hypertension, diabetes, and Sickle Cell eye disease.

Basically, the eye diseases that have the closest association with the Black population, have been mentioned. If any of these symptoms or conditions exist, go to the ophthalmologist for proper treatment, hopefully to decrease this high incidence of blindness that one is seeing in the Black population. It is important to note that secondary to glaucoma, diabetic retinopathy, hypertensive retinopathy, sickle hemoglobinopathies can all be brought under control. Each one of these conditions should be understood, and one should know how they may lead to serious eye problems.

DIABETES AND
ISCHEMIC EYE DISEASE

Diabetes causes ischemia because it causes plaque deposition. The same way it causes plaque deposition to occur within the vessel of the legs, (causing narrowing), it causes plaque deposition of the vessels of the eye. When these delicate vessels have plaque deposition, and platelet deposition, occlusion develops. The occlusion causes hemorrhage and rupture leading to different types of diabetic retinopathy. (That is basically the underlying pathophysiology as to why these three conditions occur and why they lead to blindness.)

The eye, of course, is the only organ in the body where one can actually see a vessel with the naked eye by using an ophthalmoscope. It is very important that all referrals by the physician are made to an ophthalmologist, who is well equipped to provide the appropriate treatments for patients with eye problems.

OPTHALMOLOGISTS
AND OPTOMETRISTS

There is a difference between ophthalmologists and optometrists. An ophthalmologist is an individual who is highly trained and highly equipped to provide the appropriate medical care. The optometrist deals basically with glasses, filling out prescriptions that the ophthalmologist writes. There is a big difference. If your eyes have not been examined properly by an ophthalmologist, then there hasn't really been an eye exam, you may have had your glasses adjusted, your prescription filled, etc., but the real problem with the eye is not being addressed. The ophthalmologist must prescribe the necessary medications or provide the highly sophisticated care that is needed in diabetic retinopathy, hypertensive retinopathy and sickle cell retinopathy. It is very important that this is understood because otherwise one may be going to the wrong specialist for care for too long a time. And, by the time one sees the right specialist, which is the ophthalmologist, it may be too late.

Both opticians and optometrists are experts in their own field and provide a much needed service to the public. But, an optician is an individual who has a specialty in being able to make glasses and adjust glasses as prescribed by the ophthalmologist. The opthalmologist is a physician whose job it is to examine your eyes properly. The ophthalmologist has graduated from medical school and is a specialist in diseases of the eye. It is very important that this point is made clear.

SYPHILIS AND EYE PROBLEMS

In the latter stage of syphilis, a variety of different eye problems can occur. One problem may be the small, irregular pupil that sometimes reacts to accommodation but does not react to light. Another problem might be the so-called "Argyll Robertson pupil", (the result of atrophy of the iris), which is seen in neurosyphilis. It is interesting to note that the incidence of neurosyphilis is seen three times more in Caucasians than it is in Blacks. And, neurosyphilis is twice as common in men as it is in women. Also, there are: iritis, photophobia, and retinitis. These can all be seen in secondary syphilis. There are also adhesions of the iris to the lens which can cause a fixed pupil. These problems can be detected by an internist, and then an appropriate referral should be made to the ophthalmologist. Appropriate treatments for neurosyphilis are to be started according to the Center for Disease Control. A spinal tap, (send the CSF for VDRL), and if it's positive then treat the problem with ten to twenty million units of aqueous penicillin daily (for ten days). Then, according to the Center for Disease Control, prescribe a three week course of 2.4 million units of Bicillin for a total of 7.2 million units. If the patient has a HIV infection and a positive blood VDRL, the same applies even if the CSF is negative. This is because neurosyphilis is quite prevalent in people infected with AIDS. Also, there is a high degree of false negative tests, so again, patients should be treated aggressively with ten to twenty million units of Penicillin daily for ten days; then, 7.2 million units of Bicillin to be administered for a total of three weeks.

If the patient is allergic to Penicillin, then Erythromycin, 2 grams daily (for thirty days) or Tetracycline, 2 grams daily (for thirty days) should be prescribed.

GLAUCOMA AND THE EYE DISEASE

There are three different types of glaucoma: 1) primary open angle glaucoma, 2) angle closure glaucoma, 3) (the least common form) low tension glaucoma. There are about two million reported cases of glaucoma in the United States. Glaucoma is the third leading cause of eye problems leading to blindness in the white population, and it is the first leading cause of blindness in Blacks. The incidence of blindness as a result of glaucoma is seven to eight times higher in Blacks than in Whites. In Blacks, between the ages of forty-four to sixty-five, those who have hypertension and a family history of glaucoma, have a fifteen to seventeen times greater possibility of developing glaucoma than Whites. According to published reports, glaucoma can be genetically transmitted. Thirty percent of glaucoma patients will have a family history of glaucoma.

OPEN ANGLE GLAUCOMA

The open angle glaucoma is responsible for more than ninety percent of all cases of blindness due to glaucoma. It is reported that angle closure glaucoma occurs mostly in individuals who are far sighted and are above age fifty-five. Primary open angle glaucoma is the most difficult to detect early. The first sign of this condition is when the patient begins to lose peripheral vision. Sometimes, the patient is not even aware that they have a problem until they are examined. Glaucoma is diagnosed by a test called "tonometry." This measures the pressure within the eye. Most people will have a pressure between 10 and 20 mm. of mercury inside the eye, called intraocular pressure.

LOW TENSION GLAUCOMA

Low tension glaucoma is hard to diagnose, and it has to be diagnosed by an opthalmologist. The ophthalmologist should be very astute to diagnose any abnormality in the optic nerve when it occurs. According to expert ophthalmologists, it occurs more often in the elderly and in people who have other problems with their circulation or vascular disease.

The rate of blindness as a result of glaucoma is eight to ten times higher in Blacks than it is in Whites. The reason for this is because Blacks have such a high incidence of hypertension and also such a high incidence of diabetes. Both these conditions predispose them to the development of glaucoma.

SECONDARY GLAUCOMA

Secondary glaucoma is frequently associated with trauma to the eyes. Angle closure glaucoma is less common than open angle glaucoma; but it develops very fast. The intraocular pressure rises very fast, and it causes eye pain with redness in the eye and blurry vision. If not treated quickly, the vision in the eye can be lost rapidly. Congenital glaucoma sometimes is not diagnosed until the first year of life when it is discovered that there is rising intraocular pressure in the eye. The incidence of glaucoma rises significantly after age seventy. It is also worth noting that the disease occurs in Blacks at a younger age than it occurs in Whites. The basic abnormality in glaucoma is the inability of the aqueous humor (a type of fluid that is found in the eyes) to circulate properly. Because of this, there is a back-up of this fluid in the eye, which increases pressure in the eyes because this fluid has become static.

DIFFERENT TREATMENT MODALITIES IN GLAUCOMA

Different types of abnormalities can occur in the eyes resulting in increased pressure-causing problems with the optic nerve. Once the fibers of the optic nerve are dam-aged, it is usually irreversible, which leads to loss of vision. Treatment of open angle glaucoma, usually with eye drops, and sometimes laser therapy, may be necessary to resolve the problem. It is the opinion of some experts that the success of surgery in open angle glaucoma is now as high as 80%. Angle closure glaucoma is most commonly treated with laser iridectomy, and the success rate is said to be from 85 to 90%.

MEDICATIONS USED IN THE TREATMENT OF GLAUCOMA

Some of the medications used in glaucoma are:

1. Pilocarpine Hydrochloride
2. Carbachol
3. Physostigmine Salicylate
4. Demecarium Bromide (Humorsol)
5. Acetazolamide (Diamox)
6. Isoflurophate (Floropryl)
7. Timolol Maleate (Timoptic)
8. Btaxolol Hydrochloride (Betoptic)

How to use these medications and different percent concentration is left to the discretion of the physician.

CARDIAC SIDE EFFECTS OF GLAUCOMA MEDICATIONS IN THE ELDERLY

Many of the individuals with glaucoma are elderly and therefore also have concometant cardiac diseases. So, it is important to keep in mind that these medications outlined above have systemic manifestations which can worsen underlying cardiac problems. In particular, the beta andrenergic blocking agent and non-selective beta blockers (such as Timolol) slow the heart rate. If the heart rate is slowed down too much below (i.e. 40 beats per minute or less) the elderly may not be able to perfuse his or her brain, leading to strokes; also, a similar problem can lead to angina pectoris, congestive heart failure and possible a heart attack with catastrophic consequences.

In summary, eye disease is very common in Blacks, for the reasons outlined in this chapter such as the high incidence of diabetes, hypertension and trauma to the eyes of black workers who do menial work. All of this contributes to making the incidence of glaucoma higher in Blacks than it is in Whites. Glaucoma is more virulent in Blacks than it is in Whites and the reasons are not altogether clear. Blacks not only have a high incidence of glaucoma, but they also have a higher incidence of eye diseases such as hypertensive retinopathy, hemoglobinopathy associated with eye diseases, trauma associated with eye diseases, including cataracts.

The overall economic and educational situations of Blacks will have to be improved drastically if one expects to make an impact in decreasing the accelerated rate of blindness that Blacks are suffering from.

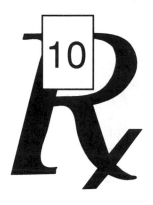

SEXUALLY TRANSMITTED DISEASES

Sexually transmitted diseases are diseases that are transmitted during sexual intercourse.

THE DIFFERENT TYPES OF SEXUALLY TRANSMITTED DISEASES

They are as follows:

1. Gonorrhea
2. Chlamydia
   a. Non-gonorrheal urethritis
3. Syphilis
4. AIDS (HIV Type I and II Infections)
5. Trichomona Vaginalis
6. Genital Herpes
7. Hepatitis B and C Viruses
8. Mucopurulent Cervicitis
9. Gardnerella Vaginalis
10. Lympho-granuloma Venereum (LGV)
11. Chancroid
12. Granuloma Inguinale
13. Giardia Lamblia
14. Entamoeba Histolytica
15. Human papillamavirus (Venereal Wart)

The Number of Published Cases of Sexually Transmitted Diseases

According to the latest published statistic by the Center for Disease Control on sexually transmitted diseases for the years 1981 to 1988 (published 12/13/89)

1. a total of 1.5 million cases of gonorrhea
2. 110,000 cases of syphilis
3. 4 million cases of chlamydia
4. 500,000 to 1,000,000 cases of human papilloma virus
5. 4,000,000 cases of genital herpes
6. 3,000,000 cases of Hepatitis B, sexually transmitted
7. 1.2 million cases of non-gonococcal urethritis
8. one million cases of mucopurulent cervicitis

9. AIDS (206,000 as of December 31, 1991.)
   The world wide incidence of AIDS is 418,403 as of December 31, 1991.

These diseases have no boundary, they can affect anyone who is involved in sexual activity. One can become infected if the person you are having sexual relationship with is infected, and you are not using prophylaxis (a condom).

GONORRHEA

This is very serious infection. Gonorrhea sometimes can become acute gonorrhea with joint inflammation (there can also be pericardial disease as associated with pericarditis, and diffuse polyarthritis associated with gonorrhea). If the diagnosis is not made quickly and the right medication is provided, the individual will risk losing the joint of the knee or an elbow as a result of acute gonorrheal arthritis. Recurrent gonorrhea not only increases the risk of having other organs affected, but it affects the gland penis which may develop urethral strictures. After recurrent gonococcal or recurrent non-gonococcal urethritis and because of strictures, a man (age fifty or sixty) can no longer pass urine. A tube has to be placed into the top of his bladder to enable him to urinate because he has destroyed his urethra. Based on statistics (1981–1988) as published by the Center for Disease Control, in 1988 there were 118,095 total cases of gonorrhea among the white population:

54,940 men
63,155 women

118,095 total cases reported.

As for the Blacks there were 560,235 total cases of gonorrhea reported:

335,241 men
224,994 women

560,235 total cases reported.

As for the Hispanic population, there were a total of 35,239 cases of gonorrhea reported in 1988:

23,401 men

12,038 women

35,239 total cases reported.

WHAT IS GONORRHEA?

Gonorrhea is a gram negative bacterium. It is a gram negative rod that has been in existence for many years. It hides in the creases and orifices of the female genital organs and especially in the vagina. It also hides in the prostate area of the man. Based on an article (*New England Journal of Medicine,* Vol.290: No. 3, January 17, 1974, by Dr. H. Handsfield) a man can carry chronic gonorrhea, meaning that he can carry the gonorrheal organism without having any symptoms. And, every time the man ejaculates unprotected during sexual intercourse, he will infect the woman. It used to be thought (wrongfully so) that only women can carry chronic gonorrhea. The woman, in turn, after getting the infection, can pass the organism back to the man with whom she is having intercourse. And, if the same man and woman are having a relationship and the man is asymptomatic, he is going to keep re-infecting the woman. She will have vaginal discharge, pain, and chronic pelvic inflammatory disease until she is treated properly. And, until he is treated, she is going to continue to become re-infected no matter how many times she is treated. An article (*JAMA* Vol.262: No. 18, Nov. 10, 1989, by Dr. M. Shafer) describes a urinary leukocyte screening test for asymptomatic chlamydia and gonococcal infection in a male, so it is now believed that men carry both chlamydia and gonorrheal infections asymptomatically. These tests are described so that particular conditions can be detected in the doctor's office or in the laboratory. If appropriate meas-

ures can be undertaken to treat these individuals, hopefully they will discontinue re-infecting their sexual partners.

CHRONIC STAGE OF GONORRHEAL INFECTION IN MEN AND WOMEN

Both men and women can be carriers of chronic gonorrhea without any symptoms and they are both capable of re-currently transmitting this infection to their sexual partners.

WHAT IS URETHRITIS?

Urethritis is a condition when a man has had sexual intercourse with an infected woman, and starts to feel a burning sensation when urinating (after four to seven days). He will have tenderness in the groin, the glands in the side of the groin will start swelling, and he will have a thick yellow discharge from his penis, if it is caused by gonorrhea. If it is non-gonorrheal urethritis, it is likely to be a lesser yellow discharge, and it may be less copious. Sometimes, the discharge may be whitish mixed with yellow, but it would still cause burning during urination. There is still a great amount of pain, and the more frequently he has an erection, the more painful the situation becomes. He has to be seen by the doctor. If he has had sexual intercourse four days or a week prior, he will need to give this history to the doctor. Sometimes, it may happen with a woman that he has met for the first time or a woman that he has known for a while. One never knows what triggers the infection.

The recurrent inflammatory process that the urethra is exposed to during each episode of urethral infection ultimately may lead to urethral stricture causing a man not to be able to pass his urine freely resulting ultimately for the need to have an indwelling super-pubic Foley catheter inserted in his bladder for life. This scenario pre-disposes the man to the development of recurrent urinary tract infection with all its associated medical complications. It is therefore important that a man does all that he can to avoid being infected re-currently in the urethra.

TESTING FOR GONORRHEAL INFECTION

1. Gram stain of the penal discharge to look for the gram negative organism that causes gonorrhea.
2. Sending the discharge for gonorrheal culture.
3. In a woman, only the culture of the vaginal discharge is necessary because gram stain of a woman's vaginal discharge is likely to show other gram negative organisms that look like the gonorrhea organism and yet is not.

The chances of growing the gonorrhea organism is very low because the organism is very fastidious (hard to grow).

TREATMENT OF CHOICE FOR GONORRHEA

The treatment for gonorrhea is Ceftriaxone, 250 mg IM or Doxycycline. The dose for Doxycycline is 100 mg twice a day for ten days. If the patient is allergic to penicillin, he/she should be treated with Tetracycline, or if the woman is pregnant, she should be treated with Erythromycin. The dose prescribed for Tetracycline should be 1.5 gm by mouth (followed by 500 mg four times a day for four days). The dose of Erythromycin should be 500 mg (four times a day for ten days). But, there is an incidence of Tetracycline resistant gonorrhea, and in this case Ceftriaxone would be more effective.

The gonorrhea can also be treated with a newly approved medication Floxin (ofloxacin) and this medication is effective for gonorrheal and chlamydial infections. The dose for this medication for acute uncomplicated gonorrhea is a single dose of 400 mg

by mouth and for cervicitis/urethritis due to chlamydial infection and gonorrheal infection, the dose is 300 mg twice per day for seven days.

The infected individual should not have any sexual relationships until there is a revisit to the doctors' office to make sure that the discharge has disappeared. Also, the sexual partner must see a physician to be examined, evaluated, and treated as someone who has been exposed to the infection. Also, two to three weeks later, blood has to be drawn to test for syphilis because these infections usually come in *two's* and *three's*. And, eight to twelve weeks later, blood must be drawn again to test for HIV Type I infection. This is because the incidence of this infection is now quite high in individuals who have sexually transmitted diseases.

IN HOSPITAL TREATMENT OF DISSEMINATED GONORRHEAL INFECTION

Frequently, the treatment of gonorrhea becomes quite a complex treatment because one may have gonorrheal infection of the throat, the anus and different joints. Appropriate culture can be taken from the throat and the anus. And in the case of a swollen joint, the joint ought to be tapped and the fluid examined for cell count protein and sent for gram stain and culture.

The threat to the loss of a joint secondary to GC is real and can occur if the diagnosis is not made promptly and treatment started immediately. Blood cultures must be sent and x-rays of the involved joint must be taken. The treatment of choice is Ceftriaxone 2 grams IV every 24 hours for 10 to 14 days. Another excellent medication is Claforan 2 grams IV every 8 hours times 10 to 14 days. If the patient is allergic to penicillin, the treatment is Tetracycline 500 mg IV every 6 hours times 10 to 14 days.

More than 2 grams IV of Tetracycline/day ought not to be given because it can lead to liver diseases at a higher dose.

CHLAMYDIA

Since 1990, it is believed that there are six million cases of chlamydial infection affecting both men and women in this country.

Chlamydia infection in the man is reasonably easy to diagnose because the man will have a discharge which is somewhat yellowish and waterish. But, these organisms are very difficult to culture, and one must rely on the personal history of the patient. Also, there can be a chronic stage of chlamydial infection (as described in *JAMA,* November 10, 1989) and tests are now being developed to diagnose both chronic gonorrhea and chronic chlamydial infections. This chronic stage of chlamydia becomes asymptomatic in a man. And, every time that he ejaculates he is passing the chlamydial organism into the woman. Then, the woman develops a vaginal discharge which can lead to an acute Pelvic Inflammatory Disease syndrome. If the woman is not treated accurately and properly, the consequences may be the destruction of the fallopian tubes (inability to have children).

NON-GONOCOCCAL URETHRITIS

According to the Center for Disease Control, there were 500,000 reported cases of non-gonococcal urethritis in men in 1988. This is a very high number, and yet, it is probably not accurate, because not all of the cases are reported to the Center for Disease Control. The non-gonococcal urethritis is caused by the chlamydia organism. It presents itself acutely in the man with a discharge. If the woman is infected with the chlamydia organism, then the woman gets an acute purulent of discharge. Also, this leads to acute Pelvic Inflammatory Disease and tubal infection, and if not treated promptly, can later lead to spontaneous abortion. There is a 15% chance of infertility after the first Pelvic Inflammatory Disease infection, 25% after the second Pelvic Inflammatory Disease infection, and 50% after the third Pelvic Inflammatory Disease infection, and so on. Unfortunately, now one sees women in their late twenties and early thirties desperately trying to become pregnant and can't because they have had multiple bouts of infection that were not treated properly. They have been left with fallopian tubes that are scarred down with fibrosis and chronic Pelvic Inflammatory Disease with endometritis and adhesions. This is the unfortunate price for previous sexual indiscretions.

ACUTE PELVIC INFLAMMATORY DISEASE

Acute pelvic inflammatory disease with fever and abdominal pain must be treated in a hospital setting with Ceftriaxone 2 grams IV (every twenty-four hours for ten days) plus Tetracycline 500 mg by mouth (for seven days) and empirically with flagyl by mouth (three times per day). Culture for gonococcal infection and chlamydia ought to be sent to the lab before starting treatment. Flagyl is a good medication for trichomonas and many anaerobic bacteria.

Most sexually transmitted disease clinics are equipped with a general internist, and staff with infectious disease experience. It is not always necessary to have a gynecologist involved. If one has a tubal ovarian abscess and there is a question of the possibility of needing surgery then a gynocologist has to be involved to perform the surgery. But, in an office setting, a fully qualified internist is more than capable of treating sexually transmitted diseases, including acute Pelvic Inflammatory Disease and chronic Pelvic Inflammatory Disease. However, there are times when a D & C or laparascopy may be needed, and one still must see a gynecologist.

Ceftriaxone is an excellent medication, and it is good for both tubal ovarian abscess and Pelvic Inflammatory Disease. Also, it can be used in the hospital setting as well as in the office.

CHRONIC PELVIC INFLAMMATORY DISEASE

If one discovers adhesions pulling on the bowel, or a chronic Pelvic Inflammatory Disease history (they have been infected over many years by a boyfriend who has had several bouts of urethritis), then one may diagnose chronic pelvic inflammatory disease. And, unless one is very aggressive, the patient is not likely to be treated properly. Also, these patients' fallopian tubes are in danger because the tube gets scarred. When the time comes for them to have children, they will have great difficulty. Refer them to a gynecologist, but some patients (who already have gone to gynecologists without being satisfied) choose to go to a general internist. If it is a question of tubal ovarian abscess or a cyst on the ovary, they have to go to the gynecologist. But, if it is a question of pelvic inflammatory disease, a well qualified internist or family practitioner can handle this particular problem. Remember that this is not just an infection, but a sexually transmitted disease.

FLARE-UP OF PID DUE TO GONORRHEA AND CHLAMYDIA INFECTIONS DURING MENSTRUAL PERIOD

During premenstrual or menstrual period, chronic, indolent infections, such as gonorrhea, or chlamydia, tend to flare up. This may be why the man might suddenly become infected by a woman he has known for a long time. If one were to take the pus from the man's penis, culture it with an appropriate medium for gonorrhea or chlamydia, the chances of getting a positive culture are very low. These are very fastidious organisms and are very hard to grow. But, if one were to take the same pus, stain it, and examine it under a microscope, one would likely to see (in the case of gonorrhea) a gram negative rod. This is the gonococcal organism that causes gonorrhea.

THE OFFICE TREATMENT OF PID

If the patient is having symptoms such as chronic Pelvic Inflammatory Disease (PID), examine them frequently while providing prescribed treatment. If their partner is re-infecting them, instruct the use of a condom. But, unless both sexual partners are treated, the infection is going to keep recurring as a vicious cycle.

Every time the female has unprotected sex with an infected male, he will ejaculate infection into her and she will continue to have infection. She may return with vaginitis, discharge, and pain. Also, in a young woman, a pelvic sonogram must be performed in addition to the examination. One must rule out any tubo-ovarian abscess, and sometimes women may develop Fitz Hugh Curtis Syndrome (a condition causing violin band-line lesions that are pulling on the liver capsule causing recurrent lower to right upper abdominal pain.)

The best way to treat this patient is with Ceftriaxone, which is the most effective medication for the treatment of gonorrhea. However, the patient may need more than one dose of Ceftriaxone depending on the circumstances. If the patient has acute Pelvic Inflammatory Disease (PID) and acute gonorrhea, one dose is sufficient. However, chronic Pelvic Inflammatory Disease is a disease whereby there are different orifices and creases involved with the infection. It is acceptable to try treatment with Ampicillin, Tetracycline, Doxycycline and Augmentin. Sometimes, Flagyl may be added to the regimen because the Pelvic Inflammatory

Disease may not be due to gonococcal infection nor chlamydia, but rather to a whole host of other organisms that are capable of causing Pelvic Inflammatory Disease such as anaerobes, gram negative organisms such as beta hemolytic streptococcus, staphylococcus, and coagulase positive. Ceftriaxone has been available for about two to three years.

Pelvic Inflammatory Diseases—New Approach for Treatment

Pelvic Inflammatory Disease causes sever morbidity and mortality in women. The Center for Disease Control defines Pelvic Inflammatory Disease as "a spectrum of inflammatory disorders of the upper genital tract in women. Pelvic Inflammatory Disease may include endometritis, salpingitis, tubo-ovarian abscess, and pelvic peritinitis. Sexually transmitted organisms, especially Chlamydia trachomatis and Neisseria gonorrhoeae, usually are the cause, but anaerobes, gram-negative rods, streptocci and mycoplasmas have been implicated as well".

According to Willard Cates Jr., M.D., director of the division of STD/HIV prevention, Center for Preventive Services, Center for Disease Control, "In the early 1980's, we were trying to be as specific as possible about the diagnosis by hospitalizating women with symptoms suggestive of Pelvic Inflammatory Disease and using laparoscopy to evaluate whether salpingitis was present". Cates also said, "We now know that most women with Pelvic Inflammatory Disease sequelae, such as infertility, have never had symptomatic Pelvic Inflammatory Disease. These women have atypical, or asymptomatic, Pelvic Inflammatory Diseases". Based on these new recommendations from the Center for Disease Control, women who are suspected of having Pelvic Inflammatory Disease

ought to be treated early, without doing elaborate confirmatory diagnostic work-up. "If the woman comes in with lower genital tract pain, adnexal and cervical tenderness when moved, think of that as Pelvic Inflammatory Disease".

The whole approach then, as to how one proceeds in the management of women suspected of having Pelvic Inflammatory Disease, has been changed; and according to the Center for Disease Control, the new approach is as follows: "Previous recommendations have suggested that clinicians should make sure it is Pelvic Inflammatory Disease before treating. By the old recommendations, pain and tenderness would not be enough to diagnose Pelvic Inflammatory Disease. They would be looking for a fever or an increased Sedimentation rate or other measures." "Now, we are saying", states Dr. Cates, "if you have any of those signs (pain and tenderness), that's enough. This way you will get much more of a silent, asymptomatic Pelvic Inflammatory Disease." Cates stressed that "cultures and microbiologic work-up should not be discarded, but treatment should not be postponed while waiting for the results.

These new recommendations made by the Center for Disease Control are welcome and greatly appreciated by many clinicians like myself, for we have felt, since the mid 1980's, that this was the way to go and have accordingly been treating women with Pelvic Inflammatory Disease in this fashion. It is reassuring that the Center for Disease Control has now solidified our thinking by these very important new recommendations. Women will surely benefit immensely from these approaches in the treatment of Pelvic Inflammatory Disease.

SYPHILIS

Syphilis is on the rise. As of 1988, according to the Center for Disease Control, there have been 110,000 recorded cases of syphilis.

Source: *Infectious Disease News*, Vol. 4 No. 3, March 1991

Syphilis, even now, continues to be a major medical problem. It is a multi-system disease that can affect the fetus in the first trimester. The baby can be born with neuro-syphilis and other complications of syphilis if the mother had syphilis and was not treated in her early stage of pregnancy. All tests for syphilis and other sexually transmitted diseases must be done prenatally, (prior to delivery). If an infected woman plans to give birth, tests have to be performed, and the chances of the baby having contracted syphilis increases—the later the tests and treatment are completed.

THE DIFFERENT STAGES OF SYPHILIS

Primary Syphilis

In primary syphilis, one sees a chancre. A chancre is a sore, it could be on either the penis or on the vagina. Also, it could be in the throat, or it could be on the anus in homosexual and/or bisexual partners.

Secondary Syphilis

In secondary syphilis, one usually sees a rash. At this time, the person is extremely contagious because the rash is just teeming with the syphilitic organism.

Latent Syphilis

In latent syphilis, the person may not even know that they have syphilis but it is found in the blood, and in the blood it can carry into the heart, the liver, causing problems and leading 15–20 years later to neuro syphilis.

Tertiary Syphilis

Tertiary syphilis is an advance stage of syphilis which can involve the heart, the liver and other vital organs.

Neuro Syphilis

Neuro syphilis is when the disease involves the central nervous system which can cause paralysis and sometimes severe organic brain syndrome and at times insanity.

Whenever one sees a sore around the genital area, it is not always a herpes sore, it could be a syphilitic chancre. The important thing is that once this problem arises, go to the doctor and get evaluated and treated properly.

In reference to syphilitic chancres, one may actually perform a dark field and see the spirochaete that causes syphilis; in addition do the Venereal Disease Control Research Laboratory test which will take a while for the results, but one may make a diagnosis immediately by doing a dark field examination.

TESTS TO DO TO DIAGNOSE SYPHILIS

1. A dark field examination of chancre
2. VDRL (Venereal Disease Control Research Laboratory)
3. FTA-ABS (Fluorescent Treponema Antibody-Absorption)

Description of a Dark Field Examination

A dark field is a procedure whereby material is taken from chancre, placed on a slide, prep and covered with a cover slip, and is placed under a special microscope, which is darkened in a specific fashion allowing for the visualization of the spirochaetes, which are treponema pallidum. When seen, this is proof positive that this individual is infected with treponema pallidum disease causing organism; which could be either syphilis, yaws and penta.

Description of VDRL

VDRL is the routine screening test that is done for syphilis.

Description of FTA-ABS

FTA-ABS is the confirmatory test done to determine whether someone has syphilis or not based on a positive VDRL test.

OTHER NON-SYPHILITIC TREPONEMAL ORGANISMS

    a.   Yaws
    b.   Penta

The Venereal Disease Control Research Laboratory test and fluorescent treponema antibody-absorption are both positive in Yaws and Penta. These diseases are caused by spirochaetes that are similar to the treponoma pallidum which is the causative organism for syphilis. It is important to realize that individuals who come from the tropical climates of the world where yaws and penta are prevalent, maybe found to have both positive VDRL and FTA-ABS blood test and yet don't have syphilis.

In addition to this, there are false biological positive for the Venereal Disease Control Research Laboratory test that is seen in rheumatoid arthritis, lupus, and other conditions that have high gammaglobulin, but in this setting the fluorescent treponema antibody-absorption is always negative.

THE EFFECTS OF UNTREATED SYPHILIS ON THE HUMAN BODY

Syphilis is a deadly disease if allowed to go untreated. It will lead to increase incidence of death in the infected individuals as evidenced by the shameful, disgraceful, outrageous, cruel and racist study called the "Tuskegee Study."

"The course of untreated syphilis has been studied retrospectively in a group of nearly 2,000 patients with primary or secondary syphilis diagnosed clinically, before the dark field and Wassermann tests came into use (the Oslo Study, 1891–1951; and prospectively in 431 Negro men with seropositive latent syphilis of three or more year's duration (the Tuskegee Study, 1932–1972)."

"The Tuskegee Study showed that the death rate of syphilitic Negro men, 25 to 50 years of age, was 17 percent greater than in nonsyphilitics, and 30 percent of all deaths were attributable to cardiovascular or central nervous system syphilis. By far the most important factor in increased mortality was cardiovascular syphilis. Anatomic evidence of aortitis was found in 40 to 60 percent of autopsied syphilitics (versus 15 percent of controls), while central nervous systems lues was found in only 4 percent. Hypertension was also increased in the syphilitics. Thus, the incidence of cardiovascular syphilis was higher and central nervous system syphilis lower in the prospective Tuskegee Study, as compared with the Oslo Study."

The Tuskegee study is a study whereby 431 negro men in Tuskegee, Alabama were purposefully used as guinea pigs and inoculated with live syphilitic organism (treponoma pallidum) for sole purpose of doing a prospective study to see the extent of the damage that the organism can do to the human body. These men, it is said, were not made aware of the fact that they were being used as guinea pigs for the study and also that no treatment was provided for them against the syphilitic organism. As a result, as can be seen above, they suffered greatly and died as a result of the devastating effects of untreated syphilis. One wonders what happened to the wives and girlfriends of these men and their children; since syphilis is a sexually transmitted disease and it is frequently passed from the mother to the unborn fetus during the primary stage of the disease.

Source: Harrison Principles of Internal Medicine, Eighth Edition, Chapter 164 page 919 to 920

The study lasted from 1932 thru 1972. The cruelty and shamefulness of this study has very few parallels in the annals of human interactions.

TREATMENT OF THE DIFFERENT STAGES OF SYPHILIS

1. Primary Syphilis/Chancre Stage (if not allergic to penicillin) 1.2 million units of Benzathine penicillin in each buttock.
2. Secondary Syphilis (if not allergic to penicillin) 1.2 million units of Benzathine penicillin in each buttock weekly times three weeks.
3. Latent Syphilis (if not allergic to penicillin) 1.2 million units of Benzathine penicillin in each buttock weekly times three weeks.
4. Tertiary Syphilis (if not allergic to penicillin) 1.2 million units of Benzathine penicillin in each buttock weekly times three weeks.
5. Neuro Syphilis (if not allergic to penicillin) Do spinal tap, send CSF for VDRL and FTA-ABS testing. If positive, admit to hospital and treat with 12 to 24 million units per day of IV Aqueous penicillin G for 10 days or 600,000 units of Procaine penicillin G IM daily for 14 days. (It is not necessary for the patient to be hospitalized to be treated with the IM regimen of penicillin.)

If the patient has HIV Type I infection, and has positive VDRL with a positive FTA, he/she will not respond to the usual dose of penicillin. They are assumed to have neuro syphilis and a spinal tap must be performed. And, they are to be treated for ten days with IV penicillin, 12 to 24 million units times ten days even if the Cerebral Spinal Fluid VDRL test is negative. In addition, the Center for Disease Control recommends three additional weekly dosages of 2.4 million units of Ben-zathine penicillin as regimen for HIV infected individuals with syphilis.

Research shows that 7.2 million units of Bicillin treats all other stages of syphilis, except for neuro syphilis.

If an individual is allergic to penicillin and he or she has early syphilis, then the treatment is Tetracycline or Erythromycin 500 mg 4 times per day for 15 days. The same medication for 30 days in advanced stages of syphilis in this setting, except in the case of neuro syphilis.

For neuro syphilis in an individual who is allergic to penicillin, the treatment is Erythromycin or Tetracycline 500 mg 4 times per day times 30 days. Tetracycline must not be given to a pregnant woman in the first trimester of pregnancy.

In Vitro Studies show that syphilis is very responsive to Ceftriaxone, therefore Ceftriaxone 250 mg IM is good treatment for incubating and primary syphilis. The only questions that remain is what is the optimal dose of Ceftriaxone that is necessary to treat syphilis and how long is that treatment necessary?

THE NEED FOR FOLLOW-UP VDRL AFTER TREATMENT FOR SYPHILIS

Follow-up VDRL test every three months is needed to see if the VDRL titer is decreasing as a way of documenting a good treatment response. If the VDRL titer fails to decrease, this could mean that the patient has not been treated appropriately or has been re-infected. Since there is no known immunity to syphilis, one can get re-infected repeatedly. The VDRL titer should disappear completely. But, sometimes it never disappears completely. But the FTA-ABS represents the antibody marker that one has been exposed to syphilis, and it will be there for life (treated or not). Every time one treats an individual for syphilis, the sexual partner must also be treated.

It is also important to do an HIV Type I test whenever one is treating someone for sexually transmitted disease. But, the patient must give permission before the test can be done.

AIDS AS A SEXUALLY TRANSMITTED DISEASE

AIDS is the most common sexually transmitted disease in the United States, and for that matter, in the world. According to the latest estimate, as published by the World Health Organization, there are close to 1.5 million HIV infected persons in the United States, and some believe that number to be close to 5 million nationally, and close to 8–10 million worldwide. As for the number of AIDS cases in the United States, there are 206,000 as of December 31, 1991, (see Chapter 10). Since the HIV virus is found in the semen in men, and in the vaginal secretion in women, anyone who is HIV infected, is, by definition, carrying a sexually transmitted disease, therefore, making AIDS the number one sexually transmitted disease in this country.

AFRICAN-AMERICAN POPULATION AND HIV INFECTION

Sexually transmitted disease is a serious problem, and it affects the African-American population disproportionately. This is not because of genetic predisposition, but because of the high incidence of IV drug abuse among the African-American population. Unfortunately the largest group of IV drug abusers in this country are Blacks and the second largest are Hispanics. There are an estimated 3 to 4 million drug abusers. So really, the minority community as a whole, (the Blacks and Hispanics) carry a high probability of being exposed to these infections. Most of these individuals are heterosexual and are eventually going to transmit the HIV Type I infection to their sexual partners. In addition to this, many of these individuals are involved in prostitution. So therefore, they also carry syphilis, gonorrhea, Hepatitis B, and chlamydia. They can also transmit herpes simplex Type II and the papillomavirus.

USE CONDOMS: SAFE SEX

The warning is for women to be careful and not to have sex with men they do not know. And, when they do have sex with someone, use a condom. Also, women who use IV drugs or are into prostitution may transmit gonorrhea, syphilis, chlamydia, human papillomavirus, genital herpes, trichomonas, Hepatitis B. They can transmit all these diseases and also venereal warts. Again, there already is a very high incidence of sexually transmitted disease in the African-American population and the Hispanic population because of the high incidence of drug abuse. 28.2% of the cases of AIDS are found in the black population, yet Blacks represent only 12% of the total population. 15.9% of the cases of AIDS are found in the Hispanic population while, they comprise only 8% of the population. 44.1% of the total AIDS cases are found in Blacks and Hispanics, and these two together represent only 19% of the total population.

People who have the HIV infection can also have other infections, such as gonorrhea and syphilis. It is important to mention that syphilis (when found in someone who has an HIV Type I infection) has to be handled differently. Although the person might appear to have primary syphilis, they will not respond the same as a normal person. Someone who has primary syphilis and who has HIV infection or AIDS has to be treated as if they have neuro syphilis. They have to receive 12–24 million units of penicillin G IV in the hospital for ten days. Because of the HIV infection, they are immuno suppressed and their response to treatment is not normal. If they are treated only for primary syphilis or secondary syphilis, they are likely to later develop neurosyphilis. In addition, HIV infected individuals must be treated with 2.4 million units of Bicillin IM in the buttocks weekly (for three weeks).

According to the Center for Disease Control, sixty-three percent of all sexually transmitted diseases occur among people less than twenty-five years of age. Two and a half million teen-agers are affected annually by sexually transmitted disease. The most serious complications caused by STD (sexually transmitted diseases) are: Pelvic Inflammatory Disease, infertility and tubal pregnancy, adverse pregnancy outcome, such as: infant pneumonia, infant death, mental retardation, immune deficiencies and neoplasia (Center for Disease Control 12/31/89). The vast majority of involuntary infertility (women who would like to have children but can't) is the result of sexually transmitted diseases. Chronic Pelvic Inflammatory Disease is probably the number one cause of infertility in women. According to the *Morbidity and Mortality Weekly Report* (February 2, 1990. Vol.39: No. 4), in 1990, the rate of gonorrhea will decrease to 280 cases per 100,000. However, among the African-American the rate of gonorrhea seems to remain stable and is not decreasing. If anything, it is stable and increasing because of carelessness and the non use of condoms. AIDS has become the major health threatening disease to the Black population in the U.S.

Most sexually transmitted diseases are treatable and curable, but AIDS is not curable. Therefore the Black community must become more aware of the ways to prevent STD such as AIDS, gonorrhea, syphilis, herpes, chlamydia, chancroid and PID. The crack epidemic may be contributing a lot to this problem. People who are on crack lose all sense of mental stability. They may be involved in risky sexual behavior and eventually they may transmit the disease. And, since most black people are sexually intra-ra-

cial, they are more likely to become infected by another black person.

It doesn't matter what one looks like, how well one is dressed or how well educated one is, if one has sexual relationship without using a condom one is exposed to the possibility of being infected. If one is married and in a monogamous relationship, the chances of becoming infected are much lower, but not nil. However, if one entered the marriage carrying the disease, the possibility of transmission is guaranteed. If one is single and having a monogamous relationship, the chances are very low, so long as one is not promiscuous, using drugs, or bisexual. But, if one is promiscuous and is involved in unprotected sex, the chances are very high. The important thing is to modify one's behavior as it relates to sex, and to use condoms.

Black males need to use condoms more frequently. It seems that black men, in general, do not like to use condoms. This is a mistake because one runs the risk of becoming infected with a serious disease, such as AIDS. If you are with a partner that you do not know well, have each other tested. Go to the doctor and have a Venereal Disease Control Research Laboratory test, a pelvic exam, cultures and pap smears.

USE OF CONDOMS AND BLACK MALES

African-American women and other Black women in this society must take a stand to educate African-American males and other Black men as to the importance of using condoms. It seems that African-American males and other Black men hate to use condoms. If the penis glans of the Black male is larger than usual, they should not use that as an excuse not to use a condom because condoms are made in different sizes. This behavior must be changed if we are to succeed in decreasing this alarming incidence of sexually transmitted diseases in the Black population.

TRICHOMONAS

Trichomonas is an infection that is asymptomatic in the man, but very symptomatic in the woman. In the woman, it causes vaginal discharge, itching, and discomfort. It's basically a sexually transmitted disease; there were three million cases of trichomonas in 1988, according to statistics published by the Center for Disease Control (December 13, 1989). When the woman has trichomonas, it can be seen in the vaginal discharge, the pap smear report, or urinary sediment. Even if the woman is treated, the infection is not likely to go away easily because it hides within the creases of the female's genital organs. So, even though she has been treated, if she has sex again with her untreated partner, she will become reinfected. The best thing to do is to try to treat both sexual partners at the same time, in order to avoid any recurrence. The best and strongest medication for the treatment of this disease is flagyl.

TREATMENT OF
TRICHOMONAS INFECTION

There were some three million cases of trichomonas reported by the Center for Disease Control in 1988. Trichomonas has to be treated by evaluating the woman and performing a pap smear. One should be able to see the trichomonas organism in the pap smear. In the man, spin some urine down and one may see it in the sediment. It may also be seen in the sediment of the woman's urine. Trichomonas causes a discharge, itchiness, and extensive discomfort for the woman. It is very important that she be treated with flagyl. She should take flagyl (500 mg three times a day) for a short course of 5 days. Treating the woman with 2 grams of flagyl, one dose, may also suffice. And she has to be told that she cannot drink alcohol while she is taking the flagyl because it may cause an antiabuse type reaction. The man has to be treated the same way (250 mg four times a day) for 7 days. To avoid this organism from going back and forth, both partners have to be treated at the same time. If the man carries the infection, it hides in the prostate area and every time the man has sex, he will infect the woman without knowing it.

GENITAL HERPES

There are probably more than a million cases of genital herpes in the USA. But, in 1988 the Center for Disease Control had only reported 500,000 to it. Herpes simplex is very difficult to eradicate from the body. Genital herpes is a painful infection that can be passed back and forth between sexual partners. The herpes infection is caused by herpes simplex. Herpes simplex is the same herpes that causes cold sores. These appear when the individual is under stress and it stays in the system for a very long time. In women, it can appear during the menstrual period, which may be a stressful time. In men, it appears when they, for example, take an examination or are under other kinds of stress. The sore tends to appear in the same spot all the time in women, either on the lips, or on the buttocks or on the vagina. In men, it appears frequently on the glans penis. It is highly contagious. It is recommended that the sexual partners refrain from having sexual intercourse when there is a flare up of genital herpes. In a woman it is very painful around the labia, the perineum, and the vagina. So, the key is to refrain from sexual intercourse until the flare-up is brought under control by medication.

Because it is very contagious, if a woman gives birth, at the time when she has this vaginal infection, the likelihood of the infant being infected by the herpes virus is very high. In particular, the eye of the infant is very vulnerable to being infected by the virus, and this can result in blindness. In this case, a Caesarean section is recommended. At times, the herpes infection is intravaginal, for example, on the uterine cervix. The woman may not know she has the infection unless she is told so by the examining physician. But, it can be cultured very easily. Also, one can do the Zank test to see the organism on the smear. With the Zank test, material is scraped from the herpetic lesions, placed on a slide and special stain is applied. Once stained, and placed under the microscope, the herpes virus is seen as an inclusion body within cells, thus confirming the presence of herpes virus.

TREATMENT OF GENITAL HERPES INFECTION

Zovirax cream is reasonably effective for treating local herpes, but also there are Zovirax capsules. Zovirax capsule (200 mg every four hours) should be used by those who have major herpes infection that reoccurs repeatedly (every other month) in major parts like the lips, the facial area, the nose, in the perivaginal area, and around the penis, and should be treated continuously (for one year). It is very difficult to get rid of this virus, and the response to treatment is slow.

Herpes simplex is not always transmitted sexually. It can be transmitted from mother to infant at the time of birth. It can be transmitted casually kissing someone who has a cold sore. Once one has it in one's mouth, it may spread anywhere else on the body, to the genital area in particular by just touching the sore with one's fingers.

Herpes simplex is the organism that is responsible for genital herpes. Genital herpes is a common sexually transmitted disease, there are now probably more than a million cases, although, as mentioned earlier, only 500,000 cases were reported to the Center for Disease Control in 1988. But, it is much more prevalent than this, most people do not want to report it, because they are rather ashamed of the problem. But there has to be an understanding between the two sexual partners in order to eradicate the organism. They both have to be treated with Zovirax. And if they understand the problem, and get treated properly, they should do very well after a year of treatment.

HEPATITIS B AND C INFECTIONS

There have been some 200,000 cases of Hepatitis B that were reported to the Center for Disease Control in 1988. Hepatitis B is found in the sperm and vaginal secretion. It is very easy for someone to be infected with Hepatitis B and not know it. Also, Hepatitis B can be transferred to a sexual partner during sexual intercourse. The organism enters the blood stream, and this can lead to clinical Hepatitis B infection leading to chronic persistent Hepatitis, or chronic active Hepatitis. This may lead to cirrhosis of the liver and often result in death. It is a very serious infection. People who are at high risk for Hepatitis B are IV drug abusers, or someone who has a disease that requires frequent blood transfusions. One must really take the necessary protective measures to protect one's self from becoming infected by these individuals. Once the infection enters the system, it (Hepatitis) becomes a major problem because there is no treatment for it. If one contracts Hepatitis B, then he/she is really at the mercy of his/her immune system. Physicians may try to help one deal with the different complications of Hepatitis B but often one becomes very sick, leading to liver failure and death. Hepatitis B and C can also be contracted through blood transfusions and blood components such as plasma. One can also become infected with Hepatitis B or C by being punctured with infected needles accidentally. Fortunately, many people escape becoming clinically sick with these viruses.

These individuals never develop jaundice, fever, or any symptoms of viral illness, and only when their bloods are tested is it discovered that they are positive for the Hepatitis B or C virus antigen, or antibody, or both, with normal liver function tests. These individuals are, therefore, carriers of the Hepatitis B or C virus, and are fully able to transmit it to other individuals via blood transfusions, and possibly sexually.

MUCOPURULENT CERVICITIS

In 1988, there were a million cases of mucopurulent cervicitis reported by the Center for Disease Control. It can be caused by gonorrhea, chlamydia, candidaalbican, and trichomona vaginalis. With this infection, try to make a diagnosis. If one is not able to establish a diagnosis, treat it empirically. It is a very painful type of infection and very uncomfortable for women. One may treat it with Ceftriaxone (250 mg) and or also add Tetracycline—if the woman is not pregnant. If she is pregnant, treat her with Erythromycin. Then, use some form of anti-fungal cream, such as monostat, sultran, or femstat. These conditions do respond very nicely to medication if treated properly.

Frequent Vaginal Infections

Frequent vaginal infections may be a sign of diabetes mellitus. Sometimes, this is how diabetes presents itself. An unexplained recurrent fungal infection should be reported to the doctor who should be astute enough to check the urine for sugar. If the urine does not have sugar in it, it doesn't rule out the possibility of diabetes. In order for the urine to have sugar in it, if one has a normally functioning kidney, the blood sugar has to be 180 or greater, because that's the renal threshold. One can be diabetic and have a blood sugar of 150 and yet is not passing any sugar in the urine. But, one could still be having a vaginal discharge on the basis of diabetes melli-

tus causing a fungal infection. So, the key is to have a fasting blood sugar with a two hour post prandial blood sugar. This is really all that is needed to diagnose Type II diabetes mellitus. The same way a recurrent rash in the groin, a rash that has no explanation, also may be the way diabetes manifests itself. The man can show signs of bilanitis (cracks in the foreskin of the penis) or physmosis (swelling and inflammation of the foreskin of the penis) due to fungal infection. This, too, may be the first sign of diabetes mellitus.

GARDNERELLA VAGINALIS INFECTION AND ITS TREATMENT

Another organism that causes infection is gardnerella vaginalis. This responds to either Ampicillin (500 mg BID) for five to seven days or flagyl (500 mg BID) for five to seven days.

LYMPHOGRANULOMA VENEREUM (LGV)

Lymphogranuloma Venereum (LGV) is a sexually transmitted disease caused by chlamydia and trachomatis.

Treatment of LGV

The treatment of LGV is Tetracycline 500 mg QID times 10 days or Erythromycin 500 mg times 10 days.

CHANCROID

Chancroid is caused by hemophylis ducreyi. It has a 4–5 days incubated period and causes vesiculo-postular lesions in the gland penis or around the labia in the woman with ulceration.

Treatment of Chancroid

The treatment for Chancroid is Tetracycline 500 mg QID times 10 days.

GRANULOMA INGUINALE

Granuloma Inguinale is caused by organism containing Donovan body. It causes pimples and ulcers on the penis of men and around the labia of women infected with it.

Treatment of Granuloma Inguinale

The treatment for granuloma inguinale is tetracycline 500 mg QID times ten days.

GIARDIA LAMBLIA

Giardia Lamblia is a protozoa that can be transmitted sexually via anal intercourse resulting in severe diarrhea.

Treatment of Giardia Lamblia

Treatment of Giardia Lamblia is flagyl 500 mg QID 4 times a day times 10 days.

ENTAMOEBA HISTOLYTICA

Entamoeba Histolytica is an organism that can be transmitted via anal intercourse and can cause severe diarrhea and/or liver abscess.

Treatment of Entamoeba Histolytica

The treatment for entamoeba histolytica is flagyl 500 mg QID 4 times a day times 14 days.

PAPILLOMAVIRUS (VAGINAL WARTS)

Over a million cases of Papillomavirus were reported in 1988 to the Center for Disease Control. Papillomavirus (venereal warts) is very common. Sixty percent of those who have venereal warts and have intercourse without using a condom, infect their partners.

Treatment of Papillomavirus

Unfortunately, there is no definite treatment for this condition. There are many procedures that have been attempted such as: currettage, surgical excision, liquid nitrogen, dry ice, and local application of 25% podophyllum tincture. There is a very corrosive type of procedure, but it has worked in some cases. However, it is very difficult to get rid of venereal warts, and they are dreadfully contagious. In the female, they can become a major problem in the area around the vagina. In the male, they ar found on the head of the foreskin of the penis; they are also found on the anus. If they bleed, they cause severe discomfort and pain.

CANCER ASSOCIATED WITH SEXUALLY TRANSMITTED DISEASES

There are cancers that are known to be associated with sexually transmitted diseases and chronic inflammatory disease such as: anal cancer (as seen in human papillomavirus), Carcinoma of the cervix (commonly seen in association with chronic pelvic infection) and associated cervical infection. The recurrent infection of the uterine cervix damages the cervical tissues to a point where these cells transform from normal to abnormal cells which then can evolve into different grades of cervical cancer. From cancer in situ all the way to aggressive cervical cancer. The causes of cervical cancer are many, but chronic and recurrent cervical infection is one of them. Cancer of the penis, (associated with recurrent penal infections) and liver carcinoma can be associated with Hepatitis B infection (sexually transmitted). Kaposi's Sarcoma is associated with the HIV infection and HIV Type I infection because the sperm carries HIV-I virus, and it is also carried in vaginal secretions.

CANCER OF THE CERVIX IN THE BLACK POPULATION

There is a higher incidence of cancer of the cervix among the black population. Because there is an association between cervical cancer and recurrent vaginal infection;

decreasing the incidence of infection could cut down on the incidence of cervical cancer.

CANCER OF THE CERVIX AND EARLY SEXUAL INTERCOURSE

Recurrent Vaginal Infection and Cancer of the Cervix

The cervix is a very delicate tissue, and the more it gets irritated through frequent sexual activity, (especially sex at an early age), and frequent infections, the more the tissue become dysplastic. The chances increase for the development of an abnormal pap smear. Also, the more it is exposed to these abnormal sexually transmitted viruses, the more likely it is to become cancerous. It seems that when women have a vaginal discharge, there is a tendency to buy and use pretty corrosive douches (such as vinegar or lysol). This is very self-destructive and very dangerous. This can make the situation worse. There are certain bacteria and fungi that live in the vagina as part of the normal habitat. If one has a vaginal discharge, go to a physician and have it evaluated and treated properly. Bacteria and the fungi live in the vagina on the check and balance system. If one kills the bacteria, the fungi will grow uninhibitedly and may cause another vaginal discharge due to fungus. Therefore, douche with just clear water after the menstrual period to remove the excess blood. That is all that is necessary.

CANCER OF THE CERVIX AND MULTIPLE SEXUAL PARTNERS

The more sexual partners, the more frequent infection, the higher the possibility of cancer of the cervix. This is a known fact, so therefore, one should be careful, refrain from having multiple sexual partners, and refrain from having recurrences of cervical infections. This will then decrease one's chance of developing cervical cancer. Plus, it is impor-

tant to have a pap smear performed once a year. If an abnormal pap is discovered make sure that treatment is begun quickly. Bear in mind that the younger the woman starts having sexual intercourse, the higher the likelihood that cervical cancer may develop in the future. Again, the more sexual partners, the more probability for developing cancer of the cervix.

SPHEGMA

Sphegma is a substance that is found underneath the foreskin of the glans penis of a man who is not circumcised. One has to be very careful only to have intercourse with a man who is basically very clean. If sphegma comes in contact with the cervix because the man is not clean, again one is likely to be predisposing one's self to cancer of the cervix. Sphegma has been known to cause cancer when placed in the skin of a laboratory animal. Men who are not circumcised are not all carrying sphegma that can cause cancer of the cervix. But because of sphegma, if the foreskin is not cleansed properly, it can cause problems for the women. There is nothing wrong with having intercourse with a man who is not circumcised. Most men in the third world are not circumcised, and yet there is not an epidemic of cancer of the cervix. One has to clarify that, but also to be complete one must mention sphegma and its possible problems.

CANCER OF THE CERVIX AND HIV INFECTION

Recently it has been discovered that a very aggressive form of cancer of the cervix is found in women who have either HIV infection or full blown AIDS. It is believed that this sub-group of cervical cancer is associated with the HIV infection in some unknown manner, yet to be determined. Therefore, every woman who is HIV infected must have frequent cervical pap smears, preferably every six months, in order that this cancer can be detected in its earliest form.

SUMMARY

In summation, the problem of sexually transmitted disease is one that can be eradicated by a change of behavior and sexual habits within society. This change in behavior should be implemented early in junior high school, so that teen-agers can become better informed of the means of protecting themselves against these diseases. Sex education classes can indirectly prevent these infections before they begin by teaching preventative methods. Because the long term complications are so devasting, it is most imperative to prevent them from occurring. Also, the Black population must be exposed more to the media, books, articles (written in popular magazines) that inform about these diseases. Also, listen to lectures that are given by people who are expert in this field. Hopefully the black community can learn how to protect itself and how to prevent all these chronic infertility problems resulting from chronic pelvic infections. So, the black community must learn to protect itself from these diseases so it can eventually eradicate their horrible consequences, and in doing so, ensuring itself of less suffering and a healthier future.

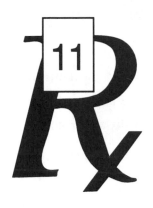

AIDS (ACQUIRED IMMUNE DEFICIENCY SYNDROME)

BEGINNING OF THE AIDS EPIDEMIC

In 1981, an article was published in the *New England Journal of Medicine* describing a new syndrome in a group of homosexual men whose immune system was found to be depressed. They were infected by bizarre micro-organisms, such as Pneumocystis Carinii and different types of fungi. These infections were leading to their death. This was the first published report of the beginning of the AIDS epidemic. According to the Center for Disease Control, as of December 31, 1991, there are a total of 206,000 reported cases of AIDS in the United States. Of this number—more than 60%, 133,000 have already died of the disease. The worldwide number of AIDS cases, as published by the World Health Organization, as of June, 1991, is 418,403.

THE NUMBER OF HIV INFECTED PEOPLE IN THE AMERICAN POPULATION

The number of people who are infected by the HIV virus in the American population is anywhere from one and a half million to six million. The worldwide statistics are anywhere from eight million to ten million.

THE NUMBER OF HIV INFECTED PEOPLE WORLD WIDE

FUTURE HIV INFECTION

"The World Health Organization estimates that 8–10 million adults and 1 million children worldwide are infected with human immunodeficiency virus (HIV), the etiologic agent of AIDS. By the year 2000, 40 million persons may be infected with HIV (3). More than 90% of these persons will reside in developing countries, in sub-Saharan Africa, South and Southeast Asia, Latin America, and the Caribbean. In addition, during the 1990's, mothers or both parents of more than 10 million children will have died from HIV infection/AIDS."[1]

RETROVIRUS

HTLV-I AND T CELL LYMPHOMA

The AIDS virus was originally called HTLV-III. It belongs to a family of viruses called retroviruses. The retroviruses have been in existence for a very long time. There is another virus related to the HTLV-III virus—the HTLV-I. This virus is known to cause T-cell lymphoma and is also associated with the tropical paralytic syndrome, seen particularly in Jamaica the West Indies. The incidence of T-cell lymphoma is significantly increasing in this part of the world, and also in Japan. A certain section of Japan has a high incidence of T-cell lymphoma. The HTLV-I virus is transmitted sexually. It is also transmitted via blood transfusion and blood component transmission. Therefore, the mode of transfusion of the HTLV-I virus is similar to the AIDS virus.

HTL-II AND T CELL LEUKEMIA

HTLV-III, known as the HIV Type I virus. There is another virus, which is called the HTLV-II virus. HTLV-II is the virus that is associated with hairy-cell leukemia, (a malignant type of leukemia that has worldwide distribution). The AIDS virus has now been renamed HIV-I. Since the renaming, there has been an HIV-II virus, (first reported in West Africa), which also causes AIDS.

HOW THE HIV TYPE I VIRUS ENTERS THE BODY

Blood

In order for the AIDS virus to enter into the human body, it has to come in contact with the blood of the individual. This has to be through sexual contact, blood

1. Reference: *Morbidity and Mortality Weekly Report* Vol. 40, No. 22, June 7, 1991'

transfusions, or the use of infected needles. In particular, those who are IV drug users, by sharing needles which contain blood of individuals infected with the virus, transmit the virus in this fashion.

Semen and Vaginal Secretion

Also, the virus is known to be found in the semen of men. So, if men are infected and they have sexual contact either with other men anally or with women vaginally, they can transmit the virus. During sexual contact, there is always micro-trauma that occurs due to capillary breakage. Therefore, the virus enters the tissues of the vagina because of the micro-trauma. The trauma may not be visible to the naked eye, but does occur every time one has sexual intercourse. In the case of the homosexual transmission, the anal tissue gets traumatized during penetration because it is not designed for the purposes of sexual contact. The anal tissue is not properly lined to be resistant to trauma; therefore, this tissue is traumatized very easily. Once the semen is placed within the anal aperture, the virus finds its way into the blood stream very easily—resulting in HIV infection.

Saliva, Urine, Stool, and Tears

The virus is also found in saliva, and one has to assume that through passionate kissing, there may be capillary breakage. If one just kisses someone on the cheek, it is not likely to happen, but if one is involved in deep passionate kissing, it may happen. The virus is also known to be found in the tears, urine, etc. It is definitely found in the stool. But, in order for one to be infected with a virus that is in the stool, one would have to have a cut in one's hand and be involved in cleaning, without gloves, of the individual who is infected. Any secretion is likely to contain the HIV virus, and if that body secretion comes in contact with an opening in the other person's body, then, of course, the virus can be transmitted. The most important thing to understand is that one cannot contract the AIDS virus by just living in the same house with someone, or by just sitting in the same classroom with them. The virus is not transmitted via the air. So, sitting next to someone in the classroom or staying in the same house with someone infected with the AIDS virus (using their own utensils) is relatively safe. On the other hand, intimate sexual contact with an individual who is infected, highly increases the chances of becoming infected with the virus.

HIV NUMBER OF HETEROSEXUAL AIDS CASES IN WOMEN AND MEN

The total number of the heterosexually transmitted HIV Type I infection in men leading to AIDS in the United States, as of February, 1991, is 3,553 as reported by the Center for Disease Control. Of that number, 606 cases occurred in white males, 2,558 occurred in black males, 373 cases occurred in Hispanic males, and 11 occurred in others.

The total number of heterosexually transmitted HIV Type I infection in women leading to AIDS in the United States as of February, 1991, is 5,354 as reported by the Center for Disease Control. Of that number, 1,294 cases occurred in white females, 2,755 occurred in black females, 1,250 cases occurred in Hispanic females, and 37 cases in other females.

KNOWN ROUTES OF TRANSMISSION OF THE AIDS VIRUS

Inoculation of blood
Transfusion of blood and blood products
Needle sharing among intravenous drug users
Needle stick, open wound, and mucous membrane
Exposure in health care workers
Injection with unsterilized needles

Sexual

Homosexual (male to male)
Heterosexual (male to female and female to male)

Perinatal

Intrauterine
Peripartum

ROUTES INVESTIGATED AND NOT SHOWN TO BE INVOLVED IN TRANSMISSION OF AIDS

Close personal contact in:
> Household
> Workplace
> School
Health-care workers without exposure to blood

BLOOD TRANSFUSION AND THE TRANSMISSION OF THE AIDS VIRUS

Blood transfusion can also transmit the virus. However, before 1985 there was a significantly high incidence of HIV infection as a result of transfusion. But, after 1985, the likelihood of the blood containing HIV infection has decreased significantly. This is because; 1) the individuals who are involved in drawing blood are more careful from whom they draw blood, 2) the blood is screened very thoroughly before transfusion. It is screened by the HIV ELISA Technique. If the blood is found to be positive, the blood is discarded. But, there is a window period in which someone can be infected, and yet, the ELISA test might be negative.

THE NUMBER OF AIDS CASES DUE TO BLOOD TRANSFUSION

The total number of AIDS cases which are the result of blood transfusion, are 3,787 cases in adults, and 255 cases in pediatrics, totaling 4,042 cases, according to the Center for Disease Control *HIV/AIDS Surveillance*, March, 1991 issue. The chances of getting AIDS from blood transfusion is said to be 1 in 40,000 blood transfusions 1987.

THE ELISA AND WESTERN BLOT TESTS FOR AIDS

The ELISA test stands for the Enzyme Linked Immuno Absorbent Assay. The Western Blot is the confirmatory test used to determine whether or not the ELISA test is accurate.

HEMOPHILIACS AND AIDS

Another group of individuals who may be infected are hemophiliacs because by necessity they have to get blood components and blood. (They are also lacking either factor 8 or factor 9.) In pre-1985, there was a significant group of hemophiliacs who were infected.

The total number of adult AIDS cases in hemophiliacs as a result of blood components transfusion is 1,434, and for pediatric hemophiliac cases the number is 145, for a grand total of 1,579, according to the Center for Disease Control *HIV/AIDS Surveillance*, March, 1991 issue.

WHY THE BODY BECOMES IMMUNOSUPPRESSED

T & B LYMPHOCYTES

The body becomes immunosuppressed in HIV infection because the T lymphocytes in the body are made to function abnormally as a result of the invasion of these lymphocytes by the HIV Type I or HIV Type II virus. The T lymphocytes that are involved in HIV infection are the T helper (also known as T-4 and CD-4 lymphocytes), and the T suppressor lymphocytes (also known as T-8 or CD-8). The T-8 is a suppressor cell. T-8 suppresses the body by suppressing the immune system when its level is high. The T-4, on the other hand, is a helper cell, it is there to aid the body in having a stronger immune system. The first cell that the HIV virus attacks, when it enters the human body, is the CD-4 or the T helper cell. It destroys the cell by incorporating itself into the nuclear material of the CD-4 lymphocyte, causing its destruction, leading to a decreased number of T helper lymphocyte and an increased number of T suppressor or CD-8 lymphocyte; thereby causing an inverted ratio of CD-4—CD-8, leading to immunosuppression, resulting in the disease known as Acquired Immune Deficiency Syndrome (AIDS).

NORMAL T HELPER AND T SUPPRESSOR LYMPHOCYTES

The following is an example of a normal T helper and T suppressor lymphocyte study in a 40 year old woman.

Normal Values	Patient's
% T cells (60.1–88.1%)	80
% B cells (3–20.8%)	13
% Helper cells (34–67%)	55
% Suppress T cells (10–41.9%)	23
Lymphocytes (0.66–4.60 THO/UL)	2.5
T cells (644–2201 CELLS/UL)	2000
B cells (82–392 CELLS/UL)	325
Helper cells (493–1191 CELLS/UL)	1075
Suppressor cell (182–785 CELLS/UL)	575
H/S ratio 1 or greater	2.39

ABNORMAL T HELPER AND T SUPPRESSOR LYMPHOCYTES

Table 2. The following is an example of an abnormal T helper and T suppressor lymphocytes study in a 20 year old patient with HIV infection:

T- and B-Cell Surface Markers: T-Helper/T-Suppressor Lymphocyte Ratio, Blood		Patient's		Normal
% T Cells		75	%	60.1–88.1
% Helper Cells	L	16	%	34–67
% Suppressor T Cell	H	60	%	10–41.9
% B Cells		6	%	3–20.8
Lymphocytes		3.0	thou/UL	0.66–4.60
T Cells	H	2250	cells/UL	644–2201
Helper Cells	L	480	cells/UL	493–1191
Suppressor Cells	H	1800	cells/UL	182–785
B Cells		180	cells/UL	82–392
H/S Ratio	L	0.27		1 or greater

PANCYTOPENIA IN AIDS
PARVO VIRUS IN AIDS

HIV virus has the ability to affect not only the immune system, but also the antibody producing system, which is also needed in order to fight off infections. By the time an individual develops full blown AIDS, frequently pancytopenia develops (the white blood cell count is low, red blood cell count is low and the platelet count is low). The HIV virus, itself, has the ability to suppress the marrow, resulting in the pancytopenia. It has been reported that in the setting of AIDS, that PARVO Virus No. 19 infects the early red cell precursors, preventing the maturation of these cells into normal red cells, resulting in severe anemia.

ERYTHROPOIETIN IN AIDS

GRANULOCYTE—MACROPHAGE COLONY STIMULATING FACTOR (GM-CSF) IN AIDS

ITP IN AIDS

TREATMENT OF ITP IN AIDS

These individuals appear to respond to IV immune globulin. When it is the HIV that is responsible for the low red cell count, these patients, if they have a low level of erythropoietin, tend to respond to epogen (which is a synthetic erythropoietin). Erythropoietin is needed for the production of red cells and it is usually made by the human kidney. The low white count that is caused by the HIV infection can now be treated by recombinant human granulocyte—macrophage colony stimulating factor (GM-CSF) also called (Leukine). This raises the total white blood cell count, enabling the individual to fight infections better. The low platelet count that is caused by HIV infection is an auto-immune platelet abnormality similar to ITP (Idiopathic Thrombocytopenic Purpura-like Syndrome). It can cause severe bleeding as a result of thrombocytopenia, and the treatment is prednisone or IV immune globulin. The HIV Type I and Type II viruses affect every part of the human anatomy, exposing the individual to the development of severe infections, because the body's immune system is being destroyed, leaving the individual defenseless against micro organisms.

ACQUIRED AND NON-ACQUIRED IMMUNE DEFICIENCY SYNDROME

AIDS is an acronym for Acquired Immune Deficiency Syndrome. This implies that there are immune deficiency syndromes that are not acquired. And, indeed there are! There are individuals who are born with immunodeficiency states. These individuals are just as likely to be infected with the same type of micro organisms that affect an individual who has AIDS. There are several

AIDS PATIENTS AND THEIR IMMUNOLOGICAL ABNORMALITIES

Prevalence	Specific Abnormality
Almost always present	Low T helper lymphocytic High T suppressor lymphocytic T helper/T suppressor less than 1
	Lymphopenia Selective T cell deficiency based on a quantitative reduction within the antigenic subset designated by OKT4 or anti-Leu-3 monoclonal antibodies (helper-inducer subset)
	Decreased or absent delayed cutaneous hypersensitivity to both recall and new antigens
	Elevated serum immunoglobulins, predominantly IgG and IgA in adults and including IgM in children
	Increased spontaneous immunoglobulin secretion by individual B cells
Consistently observed	Decreased invitro lymphocyte proliferative responses to mitogens and antigens (alloantigens and autoantigens)
	Decreased cytotoxic responses by natural killer cells; decreased cell-mediated cytotoxicity (T cell)
	Decreased ability to mount a de novo antibody response to a new antigen
	Altered monocyte function
	Elevated serum levels of immune complexes
Occasionally present	Increased levels of acid-labile interferon-alpha Antilymphocyte antibodies
	Suppressor factors Increased levels of B2-microglobulin and thymosin-al[2]

[2]Source: Modified from *Scientific American* 1990

hereditary and genetic immunodeficiency syndromes. The word "acquired" means that this condition was acquired when the virus entered the body. Children who are born with HIV type infection that they acquired in utero, have AIDS because there is a connection between the infected mother and the fetus. The mother's placenta is attached to the infant, so the blood transmission of the virus occurs. Also, the infection may occur because of the mixing of the mother's blood and the infant's blood during the birthing process.

IV immune globulin. When it is the HIV that is responsible for the low red cell count, these patients, if they have a low level of erythropoietin tend to respond to epogen (which is a synthetic erythropoietin). Erythropoietin is needed for the production of red cells and it is usually made by the human kidney. The low white count that is caused by the HIV infection can now be treated by recombinant human granulocyte-macrophage colony stimulating factor (GM-CSF) also called (Leukine). This raises the total white blood cell count enabling the individual to fight infections better. The low platelet count that is caused by HIV infection is an auto-immune platelet abnormality similar to ITP (Idiopathic Thrombocytopenic Purpura-like Syndrome). It can cause severe bleeding as a result of thrombocytopenia, and the treatment is prednisone or IV immune globulin. The HIV Type I and Type II viruses affect every part of the human anatomy, exposing the individual to the development of severe infections, because the body's immune system is being destroyed, leaving the individual defenseless against micro organisms.

ACCURATELY DIAGNOSING AIDS

The situation for accurately diagnosing AIDS is not always as simple as taking a blood sample and sending it for HIV screening. At times, it becomes much more complicated.

ELISA TEST AND THE WESTERN BLOT TEST

As mentioned previously, an individual comes in contact with the HIV Type I virus when it enters that person's blood. It takes from six, to sometimes twelve weeks before a test (the ELISA test) can show the presence of the infection. Again, once the ELISA test is positive, the Western Blot test is performed to confirm the ELISA test results. The Western Blot test is an actual electrophoresis of the HIV Type I protein. Therefore, it is extremely sensitive and accurate. There are several conditions and situations that can cause the ELISA test to be falsely positive. For instance, in Africa, and other tropical countries in the Third World, where there is a high incidence of infection with malaria and parasitic infestation, the ELISA test can become falsely positive because the body has the ability to perceive these infectious agents as foreign substances, and thereby develop antibodies against them. The ELISA test can falsely react positive to these antibodies in a laboratory setting. The positive test result can cause extreme confusion and mental anguish in the individual being tested. The Western Blot test therefore, is used as a check on the accuracy of the ELISA test. Because of cost, the Western Blot test is not used as a general screening test for AIDS. To further confuse the situation, a report came out, in 1990, stating that both the Western Blot and ELISA tests were negative in a group of homosexual men and, yet, the virus was cultured from their blood using a laboratory virus culture system. So, there is a window period from the time of infection, to the time the test becomes positive. During this time, one can donate blood, have sex with someone, and have the ELISA test be negative. An astute clinician should suspect that someone may be carrying the virus even though the two tests are negative. If a T and B lymphocyte test is done with an actual count of the total number of lymphocytes (the T-4, the T-8, and other lymphocytes), then one might discover an abnormality. There will be an inverted ratio of T-4 to T-8. * (see example on page 9) However, one has to be very careful because there are other conditions that can cause an inverted ratio of T-4 to T-8 and, yet, does not positively identify the HIV infection. If the risk factor is high, and there is some suspicion that the person may be infected, but the tests come back negative, it is a good idea to do this particular test. However, if the person has acute cytomegalovirus infection, this may cause an inverted ratio. Later, the person can normalize the inverted ratio when the cytomegalovirus is no longer present. The problem is that individuals who are infected with HIV virus, are also prone to be infected with cytomegalovirus infection.

AIDS RELATED COMPLEX SYNDROME (ARC)

The amount of time required for a person to develop AIDS, from the time of infection, is usually around 5 to 6 years. However, there are reports that individuals who received infected blood 8 and 9 years ago are now developing AIDS. So, there are exceptions. The different stages of HIV infection is a very complex and a clinically difficult process. First, there is HIV infected. This is when the individual is symptom-free and yet, has tested positive for the HIV virus. The second stage is what is referred to as AIDS related complex or (ARC). These individuals usually have symptoms, such as unexplained fever, weight loss, fatigue, skin rash, oral hairy leukoplakia, oral thrush, herpes simplex, and lymph nodes enlargement (lymphadenopathy). At this point, the individual can go into full blown AIDS, which might manifest itself as persistent fever, diarrhea for more than a month, weight loss of more than 10% of baseline, etc. (see below)

CLASSIFICATION SYSTEM FOR HIV INFECTION

Group I Acute infection
Group II Asymptomatic infection
Group III Persistent generalized
lymphadenopathy
Group IV Other disease:
Subgroup A Constitutional disease
Subgroup B Neurologic disease
Subgroup C Secondary infectious
diseases
Subgroup D Secondary neoplasms
Subgroup E Other conditions

WHEN TO START AZT TREATMENT IN HIV INFECTED INDIVIDUALS

Individuals who have ARC ought to be treated with AZT. If an individual has HIV infection and his or her T helper lymphocyte drops below 500, this individual should also be treated with AZT, and a T4 of 200 or less, unquestionably, requires AZT treatment.[3]

AIDS AND THE BLACK AND HISPANIC COMMUNITIES

Blacks represent 12% of the total American population, which is somewhere around 250 million people. Yet, out of the 167,803 cases of AIDS that have been reported by the Center for Disease Control, as of February, 1991, 47,603 are Black. The total percentage of Hispanic Americans in the United Stats is 7%, yet 26,853 Hispanic Americans have AIDS. There is, therefore, clearly a disproportionate number of Black and Hispanic individuals that are infected with the HIV Type I virus. There are, of course, 91,654 cases of Whites that have the AIDS virus, as of this report, which includes both men and women. Of that number, there are 87,098 white men, and 4,556 white

3. Reference: *Harrison's Principles of Internal Medicine,* 12th Edition

207

women. Of that number, 69,482 are male homosexuals and bisexuals. For Blacks, there are 16,612 homosexuals and bisexuals, and for the Hispanics, there are 10,490 who are homosexual and bisexual. It is also important to realize that of the IV drug abusers that have AIDS, 13,653 of them are white males, and 21,052 of them are black males, and 12,125 are Hispanic males.

As for females, as it relates to IV drug abuse causing AIDS, the numbers are: 1,734 for white women, 4,822 for black women, and 1,698 for Hispanic women. What these figures clearly show is that IV drug abuse is more prevalent among Blacks and Hispanics as compared to Whites. The high incidence of AIDS cases seen among Blacks and Hispanics is due to the high incidence of IV drug abuse in these two subgroups of the American society. Please note that the number of black females that contracted AIDS secondary to IV drug abuse is four times that of white females, namely 4,822 black females IVDA related AIDS compared to 1,734 white females IVDA related AIDS.

As the AIDS epidemic expands in the United States, the subgroups that are the most likely to become more affected by the AIDS epidemic, other than the homosexual/bisexual group, is the heterosexual Hispanic and Black population, as the statistics clearly show. There is a high percentage of heterosexual black males and Hispanic males that use IV drugs, thereby exposing their sexual partners to the possibility of being infected by the AIDS virus. Most of the heterosexual Hispanic and black males contracted the HIV infection through needle sharing, thus transferring the virus from one another's blood stream. As of February, 1991, according to the Center for Disease Control, 606 white males, 2,558 black males, 373 Hispanic males, 1,294 white females, 2,755 black females, and 1,250 Hispanic females, contracted AIDS through heterosexual contact. It is clear that if the spread of AIDS

among the heterosexual population is to be stopped, then IV drug abuse has to be brought under control. Nationwide, it is estimated that there may be as many as 1.5 million IV drug abusers, and that figure, according to some, may be as high as 4.5 million. The states with the highest percentage of IVDA are New York, California, New Jersey, Puerto Rico, and Washington, DC. In New York, it is estimated that there may be as many as 600,000 IVDA's, and about 70% of those are said to be infected with the AIDS virus.

According to the New York State Department of Health: "Race/Ethnicity—Minorities are carrying an increasingly disproportionate burden of the AIDS epidemic in New York State. Of the total cases through 1990, 61 percent were Black and Hispanic (34.9 percent black and 26.6 percent Hispanic), even though Blacks and Hispanics account for only 25.2 percent of the State's population (13.9 percent Black, 11.3 percent Hispanic). Nationwide, 44.1 percent of total AIDS cases are black or Hispanic (28.2 percent Black, 15.9 percent Hispanic)."[4]

IV DRUG ABUSE AND THE SPREAD OF AIDS

It is believed that in the near future, the IV drug abuse number will pass the homosexuality/bisexuality figure, because the gay community is taking appropriate measures to control the spread of AIDS. But, in the Black and Hispanic communities, nothing is being done to control the spread of AIDS, because IV drug abusers do not use condoms. These individuals are so distraught with their problems, and so preoccupied with their drug abuse habits that they do not think in terms of protection. Often times, they sell themselves as prostitutes so they can buy drugs. Individuals who use IV drugs are not always

4. Reference: *AIDS in New York State through 1990,* published by the New York State Department of Health.

"down and out". Some of them are people who have good jobs and who move about in the community in the middle and upper classes. Some of them are working on Wall Street and they are well dressed and well educated. They are likely to pass on the infection to a large percentage of the community, because of their positions, and because they will find sexual partners very easily. As far as the "down and out" drug abusers are concerned, they are infecting a large percentage of their sexual partners, as evidenced by the statistics published by the Center for Disease Control, February, 1991. While AIDS is being controlled in the homosexual community, because of the practices of safer sex, it is now spreading to the rest of society because of IV drug abuse among the Blacks and Hispanics.

DEFINITION OF AIDS

In order for a person to be said to have AIDS, certain clinical criteria have to be met:

WHEN HIV STATUS OF PATIENT IS UNKNOWN OR INCONCLUSIVE

If laboratory tests for HIV infection were not performed or gave inconclusive results and the patient had no other cause of immunodeficiency listed in IA (see below) a definite diagnosis of any disease listed in IB (see below) indicates AIDS.

A. Causes of immunodeficiency that disqualify a disease as an indication of AIDS in the absence of laboratory evidence of HIV infection.
   1. The use of high-dose or long-term systemic corticosteroid therapy or other immunosuppressive/cytotoxic therapy within three months before the onset of the indicator disease.
   2. A diagnosis of any of the following diseases within 3 months after diagnosis of the indicator disease: Hodgkin's disease, non-Hodgkin's lymphoma (other than primary brain lymphoma), lymphocytic leukemia, multiple myeloma, any other cancer of lymphoreticular or histiocytic tissue, or angioimmunoblastic lymphadenopathy.
   3. A genetic (congenital) immunodeficiency syndrome or an acquired immunodeficiency syndrome that is atypical of HIV infection, such as one involving hypogammaglobulinemia.

B. Diseases that indicate AIDS (requires definitive diagnosis)
   1. Candidiasis of the esophagus, trachea, bronchi, or lungs.
   2. Cryptococcosis, extrapulmonary.
   3. Cryptosporidiosis with diarrhea persisting for more than one month.
   4. Cytomegalovirus disease of an organ other than the liver, spleen, or lymph nodes in a patient older than one month.
   5. Herpes simplex virus infection causing a mucocutaneous ulcer that persists longer than one month; or herpes simplex virus infection causing bronchitis, pneumonitis or esophagitis for any duration in a patient older than one month.
   6. Kaposi's sarcoma in a patient younger than 60 years.
   7. Lymphoid interstitial pneumonia or pulmonary lymphoid hyperplasia (LIP/PLH complex) in a patient younger than 13 years.
   8. Lymphoma of the brain (primary) affecting a patient younger than 60 years.
   9. Mycobacterium avium complex or M. kansasii disease, disseminated

(at a site other than or in addition to the lungs, skin, or cervical or hilar lymph nodes).

10. Pneumocystis carinii pneumonia.
11. Progressive multifocal leukoencephalopathy.
12. Toxoplasmosis of the brain in a patient older than one month.

WHEN PATIENT IS HIV POSITIVE

Regardless of the presence of other causes of immunodeficiency (see IA, above), in the presence of laboratory evidence of HIV infection, any disease listed in IB (see above) or in 11A or 11B (see below) indicates a diagnosis of AIDS.

A. Diseases that indicate AIDS (requires definitive diagnosis)
   1. Bacterial infections, multiple or recurrent (any combination of at least two within a two-to-four-year period), of the following types in a patient younger than 13 years: septicemia, pneumonia, meningitis, bone or joint infection, or abscess of an internal organ or body cavity (excluding otitis media or superficial skin or mucosal abscesses) caused by Hemophilus, Streptococcus (including pneumococcus), or other pyogenic bacteria.
   2. Coccidioidomycosis, disseminated (at a site other than or in addition to the lungs or cervical or hilar lymph nodes).
   3. Histoplasmosis, disseminated (at a site other than or in addition to the lungs or cervical or hilar lymph nodes).
   4. HIV encephalopathy.
   5. HIV wasting syndrome.
   6. Isosporiasis with diarrhea persisting for more than one month.
   7. Kaposi's sarcoma at any age.
   8. Lymphoma of the brain (primary) at any age.
   9. M. tuberculosis disease, extrapulmonary (involving at least one site outside the lungs, regardless of whether there is concurrent pulmonary involvement).
   10. Mycobacterial disease caused by mycobacteria other than M. tuberculosis, disseminated (at a site other than or in addition to the lungs, skin, or cervical or hilar lymph nodes).
   11. Non-Hodgkin's lymphoma of B cell or unknown immunologic phenotype and the following histologic types: small noncelaved lymphoma (Burkitt's or non-Burkitt's) or immunoblastic sarcoma.
   12. Salmonella (nontyphoidal) septicemia, recurrent.
B. Diseases that indicate AIDS (presumptive diagnosis)
   1. Candidiasis of the esophagus.
   2. Cytomegalovirus retinitis, with loss of vision.
   3. Kaposi's sarcoma.
   4. Lymphoid interstitial pneumonia or pulmonary lymphoid hyperplasia (LIP/PLH complex) in a patient younger than 13 years.
   5. Mycobacterial disease (acid-fast bacilli with species not identified by culture), disseminated (involving at least one site other than or in addition to the lungs, skin, or cervical hilar lymph nodes).

WHEN PATIENT IS HIV NEGATIVE

With laboratory test results negative for HIV infection, a diagnosis of AIDS for surveillance purposes is ruled out unless:

A. All the other causes of immunodeficiency listed in IA (see above) are excluded; and
B. The patient has had either of the following:
   1. P. carinii pneumonia diagnosed by a definitive method.
   2. A definitive diagnosis of any of the other diseases indicative of AIDS listed in IB (see above) and a CD4+ helper T cell count of less than 400/mm3.[5]

INFECTIOUS COMPLICATIONS OF AIDS

The number one cause of death in AIDS patients is pneumonia, specifically pneumocystis carinii. Types of pneumonia are pneumococcal pneumonia, gram negative pneumonia. Pneumocystic carinii infection (PCP) is a peculiar type of pneumonia that AIDS patients frequently tend to develop with an associated abnormality in the arterial blood gases.

DIAGNOSING PCP

To diagnose PCP one needs to perform a bronchoscopic exam of the lungs with biopsy or brushing of the involved area. The material taken from the lungs is stained and the PCP organism is looked for. Now-a-days, one can also diagnose PCP by inducing sputum from the suspected individual, using a special technique and the material taken is stained and the PCP organism is looked for. This is a preferred technique because it is

non-invasive and reasonably benign. The chest x-ray and the clinical presentation of PCP is associated with an abnormality in the arterial blood gas.

EYE INFECTIONS IN AIDS

Patients with AIDS frequently develop infection in the secondary to cytomegalovirus, which can lead to blindness.

BRAIN INFECTIONS IN AIDS

Patients with AIDS frequently develop infection in the brain secondary to HIV Type I, bacteria, fungi, protozoa, resulting frequently in meningitis. (See Neurologic Disorders Associated with HIV Infection, below)

GASTRO-INTESTINAL TRACT INFECTIONS IN AIDS

One of the most troublesome clinical problems in AIDS patients is severe diarrhea due to enteritis, and colitis associated with cytomegalovirus, protozoa such as cryptosporidium, isospora billi.

TREATMENT OF INFECTIONS IN AIDS

ZIDOVUDINE (AZT)

AZT is the most effective medication available to treat patients with HIV infection. AZT works by blocking an enzyme called reverse TRANSCRIPTASE preventing the synthesis of the HIV virus DNA. In so doing, it prevents the growth of the virus thereby preventing it from killing the T helper lymphocyte increasing the T lymphocyte's number resulting in improvement in the immune system of the individual. The stronger immune system enhances the individual's ability to fight infections. This also increases the individual's appetite and promotes weight gain and the overall well being of the individual increases. There is a significant increase in

5. Source: As published by the Center for Disease Control taken from *Scientific American* 1990

survival amongst the HIV infected individuals who are on AZT averaging in the neighborhood of three years as compared to those who are not taking AZT. The drawbacks are liver toxicity, bone marrow toxicity and severe fatigue and lassitude in some individuals. However, the biggest of all the drawbacks is the cost of this medication which averages anywhere from 8 to 10 thousand dollars per year, which means that the average working person is most likely to be unable to pay for this medication. Public assistance must be sought in order to cover the cost of this medication and other associated medical and social problems connected with AIDS. In New York State alone, in 1990, three million six hundred and twenty-nine thousand three hundred and seventy-two dollars were spent to cover the cost of AZT.[6]

OTHER FREQUENTLY USED MEDICATIONS IN AIDS

Pentamidine, Trimethoprim/
Sulfamethoxazole, Trimethoprim for PCP.
Acyclovir for herpes simplex.
Gancilovir for cytomegalovirus
retinitis and cytomegalovirus colitis.
Fluconazole, Ketonconazole, Nystatin,
Amphotericin and Clotrimazole for
fungal infection in AIDS.
Alpha Interferon for Kaposi's sarcoma.
Sulfadiazine, Pyrimethamine and
Leucovorin are used for toxoplasma in
AIDS.
Isoniazid, Rifampin, Ethambutol,
Streptomycin and Pyrazinamide are used
to treat mycobacterium tuberculosis in
AIDS.
Ethambutal, Rifampin, Pyrazinamide,
Amikacin and Cipro and used in
mycobacterium avium-intracellulare in
AIDS.

MYCOBACTERIUM AVIUM-INTRACELLULARE (MAI)

Mycobacterium avium-intracellulare (MAI) when found in the mouth or in sputum that is coughed up by a patient, probably does not cause infection. It is only when it is found in a disseminated way, such as in a bone marrow biopsy specimen, should it be considered the cause of the patient's infection leading to persistent fever. The reason is that MAI is a frequent contaminant of our water supply, resulting from bird feces, and in the normal person, it can easily be found in the mouth without causing any infection.

OTHER INFECTIONS AS A COMPLICATION OF AIDS

AIDS patients are frequently infected with the same type of community acquired infections and the same type of nosocomial infections as the result of the population, therefore, when present with fevers, and other signs of infections, ought and should be treated in the same manner as anyone else with broad coverage of antibiotics.

OTHER ORGAN SYSTEMS THAT ARE FREQUENTLY AND PROMINENTLY AFFECTED BY THE AIDS VIRUS

Skin Problems in AIDS

The skin is frequently affected by rashes of different characteristics including a psoriasis-like rash with plaques. Different types of fungal dermatitis and Kaposi's sarcoma.

Kidney Problems in AIDS

Individuals with AIDS may develop kidney disease, resulting in nephrotic syndrome with the loss of a large amount of protein.

6. Source: *AIDS in New York through 1990* as published by New York State Department of Health.

Genital Lesions in AIDS

Both men and women with AIDS can be affected with severe weeping and painful sores in different parts of the genital organs, frequently due to herpes, venereal diseases, venereal warts and fungal skin eruptions.

Joint Disease in AIDS Patients

Different types of arthritis involving the muscular skeletal system and joints have been seen in patients with AIDS.

Neurological Disorders in HIV Infection

The HIV organism has a high predilection for the brain, and the entire nervous system can be affected by it in different degrees, resulting in different types of neurological abnormalities, the severest of them are depression, organic brain syndrome and progressive multifocal leukoencephalopathy (PML), resulting in disabling paralysis. Seizures are frequently seen in patients with AIDS whose brains are affected, either by the HIV virus

INFECTIONS AS A COMPLICATION OF AIDS

	Infecting Organism	Type of Infection
Viruses	Cytomegalovirus	Pneumonia, disseminated infection, retinitis, encephalitis
	Epstein-Barr virus	Important pathogenic factor in B cell lymphoproliferative disorders and Burkitt's lymphoma, oral hairy leukoplakia
	Herpes simplex virus	Recurrent severe localized infection
	Varicella—zoster virus	Localized or disseminated infection
	Papovavirus	Progressive multifocal leukoencephalopathy
Fungi	Candia albicans	Mucocutaneous infection, esophagitis, disseminated infection
	Cryptococcus neoformans	Meningitis, disseminated infection
	Histoplasma capsulatum	Disseminated infection
	Coccidioides immitis	Disseminated infection
	Petriellidium boydii	Pneumonia
	Aspergillus	Invasive pulmonary infection with potential for dissemination
Protozoa	Pneumocystis carinii	Pneumonia, retinal infection
	Toxoplasma gondii	Encephalitis
	Cryptosporidium	Enteritis
	Isospora belli	Enteritis
Myobacteria	Mycobacterium avium-intracellulare	Disseminated infection and localized
	Mycobacterium tuberculosis	Disseminated infection
Bacteria	Nocardia	Pneumonia, disseminated infection
	Legionella	Pneumonia
	Streptococcus pneumoniae	Pneumonia, disseminated infection
	Hemophilus influenzae type B	Pneumonia, disseminated infection
	Salmonella	Gastroenteritis, disseminated infection
	Gram negative bacteria (i.e. klebsiella pneumonia, E. Colo)	Ascending colongitis
	Cytomegalovirus	Colitis
	Triponoma Pallidum	Syphilis and neuro-syphilis

Source: Modified from Scientific American 1990

itself, by infectious agents, parasitic agents, by protozoal agents, or by lymphoma.

OTHER COMPLICATIONS FREQUENTLY SEEN IN AIDS PATIENTS THAT CAN LEAD TO THEIR DEATH

Kaposi's Sarcoma
Large Cell Lymphoma

Kaposi's sarcoma, which frequently involves the skin, the GI tract, resulting in severe bleeding. For reasons that are unclear, almost always patients who have Kaposi's sarcoma are infected with cytomegalovirus. The full meaning of this is not clear but it would appear, according to some, that the CMV virus may be, in some fashion, playing a role in the development of Kaposi's sarcoma. Alpha Interferon has been used to treat Kaposi's sarcoma with limited success.

Another malignant tumor frequently seen in homosexual/bisexual males is cancer of the rectum. Large cell lymphoma is another malignant tumor that has the propensity of afflicting patients with AIDS. In these patients, large cell lymphoma is very aggressive and rarely curable, if ever.

CONFIDENTIALITY IN HIV INFECTION

The test that is prescribed to diagnose HIV infection is the ELISA test as mentioned previously. This should be followed by the Western Blot test. The test for HIV Type I can be performed in a private doctor's office,

NEUROLOGICAL DISORDERS IN HIV INFECTION

Neurologic Disorder	Prevalence (%)	Clinical Features	Histopathologic Features
Subacute encephalitis	90	Cognitive deficits, memory loss, psychomotor slowing, pyramidal tract signs, ataxia, weakness, depression, organic psychosis, incontinence, myoclonic seizures	Gliosis, myelin pallor, microglial nodules, perivascular inflammation, focal demyelination, multinucleate giant cells
Peripheral neuropathies Chronic distal symmetric polyneuropathy	10–50	Painful dysesthesias, numbness, paresthesias, weakness, autonomic dysfunction	Demyelination, axonal loss, mild inflammation
Chronic inflammatory demyelinating polyneuropathy		Weakness, sensory deficits, mononeuropathy multiplex, cranial nerve palseis, hyporeflexia or areflexia, cerebrospinal fluid pleocytosis	Marked inflammation, demyelination with secondary axonal loss
Vacuolar Myelopathy	11–22	Gait ataxia, progressive spastic paraparesis, posterior column deficits, incontinence	Vacuolar degeneration of lateral and posterior columns
Aseptic meningitis	5–10	Headache, fever, meningeal signs, cranial nerve palsies, cerebrospinal fluid pleocytosis	—
Progressive multifocal leukoencephalopathy		Brain dysfunction with paralysis	
Infection of brain, bacterial, fungal parasitic and protozoal infections		Symptoms of meningitis, fever, headache, neck stiffness	

the Department of Health clinics, or local neighborhood clinic. It is all confidential. The patient's name is not used, only a code is used. Only the doctor and the patient are aware that the test is being sent. The state has no way of knowing the identity of the patient. Besides being confidential, the patient has to sign a consent form to allow the test to be performed. The test is not performed unless the health practitioner not only has consent, but he/she is also sure that the individual is able to deal with the consequences of the results. If the person finds out that he or she is positive, the reaction has to be evaluated by the physician before the test can be performed. This is very important. However, anyone can walk into a Health Department clinic and have the test performed confidentially. What to do with the results is a very important issue. One does not want the results falling into the wrong hands. Because of the tremendous psychological impact, it may immediately affect the person's employment. Because of hysteria associated with HIV infection, there is a great deal of discrimination. People are being unnecessarily dismissed from their jobs. This is against the law. The law, now in many states and also the Federal Government, is designed to protect individuals from being discriminated against within the job force etc. It is a very, very important issue that must be kept in mind at all times when one deals with the matter of HIV Type I infection.

WORLDWIDE INCIDENCE OF AIDS

According to the World Health Organization, AIDS has been reported in 178 countries. There are significant incidences of AIDS in Central Africa, Western Africa and the total number of reported AIDS cases in Africa is 119,983. In Europe, the number is 56,227, in Central America it is 2,159, in South America it is 24,084, with Brazil having 19,361, Venezuela 1,061, Argentina 920,

Columbia 1,285, and smaller numbers in the other South American Countries. The total number of reported AIDS cases in North America is 211,116, and of that number, the United States has 206,000 (updated as of December 31, 1991), Mexico 7,170, Haiti 3,086, Canada 5,228, Dominican Republic 1,506, Trinidad and Tobago 736, The Bahamas 599, and smaller numbers in other North American countries. Also, smaller numbers of AIDS cases are reported in other smaller countries of the world.[7]

The total number of cases reported by the World Health Organization as of December 31, 1991 is 418,403. However, it is believed that the actual number is about three to four times greater. It is believed to be close to one and a half to two million cases of AIDS in the world. The figures are hard to substantiate because there are many countries that refuse to give accurate accounts for economic reasons since it affects the tourist trade. The total number of cases of HIV infected individuals who have not yet developed a serious case of AIDS in this country is believed to be from one and a half to two million, and worldwide it may be as many as ten million. Again, the accuracy is hard to determine.

AIDS AND UNSTERILIZED INSTRUMENTS

AIDS in the third world varies, whereas in the United States the vast majority of AIDS is due to homosexual/bisexual practices and IV drug abuse. In Central America, for instance, most of the individuals are heterosexual and the mode of transmission is quite different. Because of practices that are indigenous to that part of the world, individuals are being treated with intramuscular injection by practitioners that are not physicians.

7. Source: *Internal Medicine World Report* Vol. 6 No. 20 Nov. 1–14, 1991

The needles are not sterilized, therefore transmitting the AIDS virus. Some cultures use unsterilized objects to make marks on their forehead or other skin area, which is another way of transmitting AIDS. In certain parts of Africa, because of cultural and religious reasons, the woman's clitoris is removed with unsterilized instruments, another way of transmitting AIDS.

AIDS AND THE THIRD WORLD

In the beginning of the epidemic, transfusion of blood was not a common practice in Africa and there was no proper screening for the HIV infection. A positive ELISA, especially in the African setting, does not always mean HIV infection, because of infestation with parasites or malaria which give false-positive ELISA tests. Original data was published on the basis of ELISA tests that were not confirmed by Western Blot tests. Hopefully, the situation is different now that these tests have reached Africa.

Another issue of great importance in the Third World, in general, is that most men are not circumcised. A man may develop conditions such as balantitis (a recurrent inflammation of the foreskin leading to a break in the skin) or phymosis (a higher chronic grade of the same condition resulting in the scarring of the foreskin). The highest grade of abnormality is paraphimosis in terms of scarring and representing an entry point. If one has intercourse with an infected woman (a prostitute), the organism known to be present in the vaginal secretion, then one becomes infected with HIV virus. In this case the virus has to come in contact with the individual's blood. This is a highly probable way of contacting the disease. This concept was first presented by myself in an article published in the *New York State Journal of Medicine*, Vol. 86, August, 1986. There are others who seem to think that if one has a sore in the penis (associated with venereal disease) it also presents a point of entry. This is true, but venereal diseases (sores in the penis glans or the vagina) are not indigenous to the Third World. Homosexuality and bisexuality are not a common practice in the third world, but as in any case, there are exceptions. In addition, IV drug addiction is not common in the third world either, with exceptions. For instance, in Trinidad and the Caribbean, there seems to be an incidence of AIDS transmitted via IV drug abuse more than other third world countries. In Africa, IV drug use is not the modality through which AIDS is transmitted. It is also important to realize that most of the heterosexual men who were originally found to have HIV infection were very mobile. It is quite possible that the virus may have been brought back to Africa by these men when they came in contact with the prostitutes in other countries of the world, such as Europe. Polygamy is a common practice in Africa, so therefore this virus spreads through the population resulting in a high rate of AIDS in Central and West Africa. The HIV Type II virus (another retrovirus that also can cause the AIDS syndrome) was first discovered in West Africa. Sexuality seems to be the main way in which the AIDS virus is transmitted in Africa. Of course, other modalities play a role in the dissemination and transmission of the virus through the population.

AIDS AND DRUG ABUSE AND ITS EXTENT IN THE BLACK COMMUNITY IN THE UNITED STATES

Close to fifty to sixty percent of men who are in jail in this country are able-bodied black men, and of this number most of them are in for crimes associated with drugs. In New York State there were 1,388 cases of AIDS amongst the state prison inmates, as of December 31, 1990. Of that number, 188 were White, 532 were Black, 663 were

Hispanic and 5 others. 85.7% of these Blacks were IV drug users. 91.4% of this group of Hispanics were IV drug users, and 86.2% of these Whites were IV drug users, and heterosexuals. Of course racism is at the core of the problem. You have spread of AIDS in the black community because of drugs. Black folk do not have the means with which to import all these drugs into the black community. The drugs get into the black community because the majority population is involved in bringing them there. They have the power, the money, and they have the means with which to import the drugs and bring them to the minority community. Basically the blacks and Hispanics are the victims of the drug trade subculture. They are so depressed and so distressed and so stressed out that they resort to the unfortunate habit of using drugs. Drug addiction should not be condoned, it is a horrible, horrible habit. It is the worst, but one must also look beyond. How did the drugs get there? It is drugs that led to the AIDS epidemic in the black community to the degree that it exists right now. It is going to get worse and there is nothing really that is being done about it. Government is failing based on recent reports in an attempt to try to control the drug situation. They are not getting at the root cause of the problem. Namely, if you improve the lives of these individuals by bettering their economic situation, by bettering their educational situation, etc., then we will begin an advancement in this direction. There are not enough treatment centers for addicted individuals to go and get treated for their drug problems. Most are turned away because the treatment centers available to them are overcrowded.

ECONOMIC IMPACT OF AIDS 1991

$5.5 billion is estimated to be the amount of money necessary to pay for the cost of AIDS in 1991. It is further estimated that by 1994, this figure will go up to $10.4 billion per year. $85,333 is estimated to be the cost of treating one patient who has AIDS over the lifetime of that patient.[8]

CONCLUSION

It is the responsibility of the political leaders, clergy, and governmental agencies that are involved in African-American, and Hispanic communities to control the spread of this very deadly virus. Otherwise, it will run rampant through these communities. It is already becoming a catastrophe because both minority groups socialize not only with those that are infected, but are going to eventually pass the disease to those in the heterosexual community. This will only lead to the further spreading of this disease.

8. Source: *Medical Tribune*—July 11, 1991, Vol.32

.This book is useful for historical reasons only. It does not contain current medical information.